RUNNING
BREAKTHROUGHS

RUNNING BREAKTHROUGHS

Transform Your Running and Life:
Proven Lessons from World-Class Athletes,
Experts, and Recreational Runners

FLORIS GIERMAN

Copyright © 2025 by Floris Gierman

All rights reserved. No part of this publication may be reproduced, distributed, or transmitted in any form or by any means, including photocopying, recording, or other electronic or mechanical methods, without the prior written permission of the publisher, except in the case of brief quotations embodied in critical reviews and certain other noncommercial uses permitted by copyright law.

First Edition, 2025

ISBN: 979-8-9933648-2-7

Published by Floris Gierman [florisgierman.com]

Cover photo and design: Jen Gierman
Interior design by: Best Seller Publishing
Editing by: Philip Bader

This book is sold with the understanding that the author and publisher are not engaged in rendering professional advice or services to the reader. The ideas, procedures and suggestions contained in this book are not intended as a substitute for consulting with your physician. All matters regarding health require medical supervision.

The author and publisher shall not be liable or responsible for any loss or damage allegedly arising from any information or suggestion in this book.

Printed in the United States of America.

DISCLAIMER

This book shares ideas, insights and advice on health, fitness and running based on my personal experiences and interviews with experts. Please remember, everyone is different.

I am not a doctor, nutritionist or licensed health professional. The content in this book is for information only, not medical advice.

Before trying new exercises, diets, supplements or making lifestyle changes described here, talk to a qualified health professional. What works for one person may not work for you.

Use your common sense and listen to your body. If something feels wrong, stop immediately and consult someone qualified. Your health is your responsibility.

I cannot be held liable for any injuries, health issues or other consequences that may result from following the advice in this book. I realize this is a ridiculously serious way to kick off a running book. Trust me. The rest of the book is more exciting.

Stay curious, be patient with yourself and enjoy your health and fitness journey.

Dedications

To my daughters Sadie and Zoey,
begin where you are.

Keep your hearts wide open and
trust the path that calls to you.

Let wonder and joy lead your way.

run·ning break·through
/ˈrəniNG ˈbrākˌTHro͞o/

1. a noticeable leap forward in running ability, performance, or enjoyment, often after a period where progress felt slow or stagnant.

2. a transformative moment in training, mindset, or health that elevates running to a new level of ease, speed, or consistency.

3. the point where steady effort and small changes compound into lasting improvement, revealing potential beyond previous limits.

Advance Praise

From Elite Runners

Floris has this unique capacity to make conversations dive into the deepest thoughts in the most comfortable and natural way. With this book he summarizes perfectly what has driven the best athletes and coaches into excellence and how you can use that knowledge to make you a better runner and to have a healthier and more fulfilled life.

—**Kilian Jornet,** the greatest mountain and ultrarunner of all time

Being a guest on Floris's podcast was like sitting down with an old friend. His curiosity, care and passion for running and life made our conversation unforgettable. In his book, Floris weaves together powerful moments from his interviews, capturing the spirit of endurance and connection that defines the running community. It's more than a book about running; it's a tribute to the strength we find in each other's stories.

—**Sally McRae,** professional ultrarunner, bestselling author, podcast host and coach

From Health and Fitness Experts

I've been on a lot of podcasts, and I haven't met a better interviewer than Floris Gierman. Asking great questions has filled him with great answers. If you're looking for answers as a runner, read *Running Breakthroughs*.

—**Matt Fitzgerald,** bestselling author of *80/20 Running* and *How Bad Do You Want It?*

Floris is a generous, thoughtful and soulful human being who has a deep desire to help others thrive. His podcast is a masterclass in compassionate curiosity, and this book will inspire you to become the runner you have always been capable of becoming.

—**Dr. Rangan Chatterjee,** renowned physician, bestselling author and host of the #1 health podcast, *Feel Better, Live More*

Floris keeps spreading the news about breakthroughs in health and fitness. His great podcast interviews have evolved into a vast volume of invaluable information, and now he's gone the extra mile to share these running experiences in a great new book.

—**Dr. Phil Maffetone,** clinician, coach, author and creator of the MAF Method

Over the past decade, I've watched Floris Gierman pour his passion for healthy running into this book, skillfully weaving insights from dozens of the world's top experts on low heart rate training and functional movement. His dedication to uncovering and sharing practical, joy-filled approaches to running shines through, making this a must-read for anyone seeking a sustainable, fulfilling running practice.

—**Dr. Mark Cucuzzella,** a physician, professor of family medicine and lifelong runner with 25 Boston Marathon finishes

Flo is a true gem and someone I am so grateful to know. His enthusiasm for running (and life) is contagious. I met him earlier in his running career. To see him go from student to athlete, and now powerhouse coach and an endlessly inspiring podcast and content creator is just next-level incredible. His interviews are insightful and his voice authentic. I cannot recommend whatever this human creates enough.

—**Kate Martini Freeman,** Floris's first running coach

From Recreational Runners

A running book for curious running minds, *Running Breakthroughs* catalogs a lifetime of learning about endurance, performance and running. It's both a source for running knowledge and a foundation for further exploration.

—**Kofuzi,** a running YouTuber and gear reviewer

Any reader of this book will have the privilege of learning the most poignant takeaways from this treasure trove of information and inspiration. Floris has cemented himself as one of the most diversified students of the sport.

—**Eric Floberg,** a marathoner, running coach and YouTuber

There are few people I know who can match the intense dedication that Floris has to improve his running journey through thoughtful research, reflection and curiosity. Whether it's knowledge gained from personal experience or from in-depth conversations with the most elite athletes on Earth, Floris is dedicated to the constant pursuit of becoming the best version of himself. More importantly, he is passionate about sharing that knowledge with others. He does that in this book, distilling the most important lessons he's learned into something that will undoubtedly improve your own path forward, in whatever project you pursue.

—**Robbe Reddinger,** senior editor for Believe in the Run

The book *Running Breakthroughs* offers valuable lessons that extend beyond running, providing readers the tools to become stronger, happier and healthier humans. This book is a must-read for athletes at all stages of their running journey.

—**Amelia Vrabel,** running coach and marathoner

If you have become frustrated with running, or just beginning, welcome to your manual for life. Floris has taken years of knowledge and condensed it down to easy-to-understand lessons that will lead your journey. Heed the knowledge in this book. It will change your relationship with running and with life, and for the better.

—**Scott Frye,** strength, mobility and running coach

If there is any doubt in your mind, simply read this book filled with gold nuggets. This is revolutionary and successfully counters the no pain, no gain approach. I've improved from a 5-hour marathon, where I could barely stand afterwards, to 3h52 and finished dancing.

—**Todd Marentette,** marathoner and cohost of *The RUNEGADE Podcast*

From the @FlorisGierman YouTube Channel

@DP-sh3nk – Floris has genuinely shifted my perspective on running and wellness. His content is incredible! I've learned more from his content in a short time than in years of struggling alone.

@Keeniejelcabahug7151 – I suffered anxiety and depression after my dad passed away late in 2024. I started having dark thoughts, and yes, I started thinking of self-harm, and so I started walking to try and go out and appreciate the environment and the community. I started run-walk and came across your content about low heart rate training. Just want to say THANK YOU. You saved my life, dude!

@JamesMetcalf – I finally went sub 3:30 on my ninth attempt! For the first time I actually felt that I raced it instead of just hanging on for a few hours. No better feeling than overtaking hundreds of much younger runners in the 2nd half—old guys kick ass. A new PB! A big shout-out to coach Floris and his brutal Dutch honesty—you saved my race!

@JoshuaBrunner-t9k – With Floris's help, I finally broke a 4-hour marathon after 17 years of trying! I'm about to turn 50 and working towards a BQ. I especially like his interviews with everyday folks meeting, and exceeding, their personal goals.

@ChiChi1976 – I found MAF and Floris and within one week, I was off all meds. Within two weeks, I was pain-free. Before I started, I could only run 3 days a week. Now, I can run 5 to 6 days a week, and I feel like I'm 20 again. I feel great, lost 30 lbs and enjoy my runs. Also my marathon time improved from 4:55 to a 4:31.

@kirbster1977 – I've been running for ten years and struggled with injuries. Floris's insights helped me run injury-free and greatly increased my love for running again. His content is simply amazing!

@LloydGoldsteinMusic – Following Floris's channel has transformed both my physical health and my mindset. His advice turned running from a painful struggle into pure enjoyment.

@robine8192 – Your holistic approach and easy-to-follow advice made all the difference, improving my running and quality of life overall. My health and running performance have drastically improved.

Foreword

It is easier to be changed than to change.
—Robert Sapolsky

I have spent much of my life treating people. In that time, I have seen some remarkable transformations. In general, these are rare because progress is mostly slow. Personally, I was always interested in big, dramatic changes. These were few and far between. Still, it was always the big shifts or breakthroughs that inspired me and made me believe in a better way.

Floris experienced one of these dramatic and significant shifts, documented in our wonderful conversation together (extramilest.com/80). It was a spontaneous healing moment that he had been working towards, ignited in an instant of insight, healing perspective and change. He probably realized in that moment that what most of us spend a lifetime looking for is actually our birthright.

What matters for us is to find and connect with our true authentic self. This goes for movement, thoughts, insights and passions. It is our birthright and always available, but we just get conditioned, programmed and traumatized away from our true selves. It is very hard to change, but if we surround ourselves with the right resources, friends, influences and even movements and movement patterns, we can be changed in a very positive way. Mostly, it involves letting what is become revealed and expressed.

My journey into healthcare was almost certainly because my mother died of cancer when I was 11. It was the same for my brother, who later became a cardiologist. We desperately tried to save and heal those around us, so that we did not lose our rock and source of love and care in the world.

I personally had a very strong victim mentality. As a result, I was bullied when I was growing up. So my initial years as a therapist were a pretty messy affair, me being an insecure underachiever yet desperately trying to be the best at what I did. I was probably bullying people into health more than providing a safe space for them to express themselves.

Fortunately, along the way, I met role models, mentors, and had a few meaningful and life-changing conversations and interactions. Slowly, my perspective began to shift. Facing cancer myself profoundly changed my life towards a more authentic approach. Faced with the possibility of my own death or never being able to treat people again, I thought about what kind of legacy I could leave or how I could make money going forward if I could no longer treat people.

I tried to reframe what I knew from an evolutionary perspective. I began to rethink movement and what I knew about movement and posture from the ground up, rather than dwell on morbid thoughts of death, chemotherapy and possible amputations. "We cannot escape millennia of evolution" was my mindset. Now, I believe we just have to let millennia of evolution and design express itself without constraint.

It is easier to be changed than to change, and all great change happens in a safe space where we get to express ourselves authentically. Most of our frustrations are acquired from a mismatch of environment and an accumulation of programming and externalities that don't suit us. This, of course, is amplified by technology.

I no longer look at someone running or at someone's posture and point out their weaknesses and faults. Instead, I try to look at someone as whole and perfect and help create the space to awaken their original biomechanics, thought patterns and movement patterns so that they can express themselves to their fullest potential. Our best version of ourselves lies within us and is always accessible. That version is unaltered by life and circumstance, cultural narratives and opinions pulling us away from our authentic self and authentic movement patterns.

The only life worth living is a deeply authentic one, where we get to express our purpose and passion. This is where magic happens, life changes, potential gets expressed, talents and destinies open up and healing and growth occur.

The paradox is that someone trying desperately to fit in and be accepted almost certainly never will. Yet someone deeply authentic will be respected and probably accepted wherever they go.

Fortuitously, this growth, shift and change manifested when the universe bumped Floris and I together. Floris, with his kindhearted, curious and diligent approach to helping others, had an extraordinary moment of clarity, healing and self-awareness. In that moment of healing, self-love and self-acceptance, Floris was able to step closer to his authentic self and into his power and birthright, thus better able to serve his family and community, and of course, show up even more authentically.

This book is a collection of stories carefully curated and crafted together to help create the environment for change and growth. It creates the space and opportunity for new perspectives, insights and possibilities. Open up to any page or chapter, and timeless wisdom and insights are available to you from people who have powerfully connected to their authentic selves in one way or another. Floris creates a deeply authentic and safe space for guests to be seen, heard, understood, and to open up and share their deepest insights.

Floris helped me express myself and move towards my true purpose. I am sure this book will help you on your journey in the same way, too.

Lawrence van Lingen
Sunshine Canyon, Colorado

A GIFT FOR YOU!

The Runner's Breakthrough Toolkit

Access this exclusive bonus package to help you achieve your next running breakthrough:

- **Video Masterclass:** "The 3 Critical Steps for Achieving Your Personal Best" (20-minute training)
- **Race Day Success System:** Complete checklist, proven pacing calculator and nutrition timing guide
- **Implementation Workbook:** Simple exercises to translate insights into immediate improvements
- **Proven Training Schedules:** Real-world plans used to achieve breakthrough performances
- **Running Journal Template:** A structured system to track progress, build self-awareness and maintain motivation
- **Exclusive Bonus Chapters:** Additional content and advanced strategies that didn't make it into the printed edition

> Your Runner's Breakthrough Toolkit is available free with your purchase of the book.
>
> Visit **florisgierman.com/gift** and enter access code:
>
> ## personal-best

Table of Contents

START HERE: HOW TO USE THIS BOOK 1

PART 1: FOUNDATIONS 7

    Chapter 1: How to Run Longer Without Running Out of Breath 11
    Chapter 2: Start (or Restart) Your Running Journey 17
    Chapter 3: Heart Rate Training Fundamentals 23
    Chapter 4: Calculating Your Personal Heart Rate Zones 33
    Chapter 5: Implementing Heart Rate Training Successfully 49
    Chapter 6: Balancing Volume and Intensity in Training 55

PART 2: ELITE ATHLETES IN CONVERSATION 65

    Eliud Kipchoge on Consistency and Joy 69
    Courtney Dauwalter on Mastering the Pain Cave 74
    Kilian Jornet on Adaptability and Intensity 79
    Mark Allen on Mindset and Meditation 86
    Taylor Knibb on Feel over Data 91
    Ryan Hall on Strength Training 95
    Sally McRae on Mental Resilience 99

PART 3: OPTIMIZING YOUR MIND AND ENERGY 105

    Chapter 7: How to Optimize Your Energy 109
    Chapter 8: The Power of Journaling 115
    Chapter 9: Run Faster by Relaxing 119
    Chapter 10: How to Deal with Frustration in Training 127
    Chapter 11: Four Drills to Improve Your Running Form 133
    Chapter 12: How to Run a Personal Best on Race Day 139
    Chapter 13: What to Do When the Sh*t Hits the Fan 145
    Chapter 14: Yes, Older Runners CAN Still Improve 151

PART 4: EXPERTS IN CONVERSATION 157

Dr. Stephen Seiler on 80/20 Training... 160
Dr. Rangan Chatterjee on Healthy Habits 165
Dr. Phil Maffetone on the MAF Method 173
Lawrence van Lingen on Movement and Flow 180
Patrick McKeown on Breathwork 191
Kasper van der Meulen on Conscious Breathing 195
Jennifer Schmidt on Mental Health 199
Susan Piver on Meditation 203
Scott Warr and Don Freeman on Trail Running 208
Andy Blow on Hydration and Fasting 212
Kate Martini Freeman on Mindset Coaching 219
Matt Fitzgerald on Endurance Mindset 223
Kyle Long on Strength Training 227
Jason Fitzgerald on Injury Prevention 230
Dr. Mark Cucuzzella on Healthy Running 233
Matteo Franceschetti on Sleep Optimization 239
Kara Collier on Glucose Management 242
Tawnee Prazak Gibson on Holistic Health 246
Chris Hauth on Mental Toughness 250
Jimmy Dean Freeman on Mental Training 253
Amelia Vrabel on Patience 258
Scott Frye on Recovery and Mobility 261
Charlie Engle on Overcoming Adversity 264
Tim Rowberry on Sustainable Training 268
Believe in the Run on Running Gear 271

PART 5: THE JOURNEY OF THE EVERYDAY ATHLETE 277

Chapter 15: Play the Long Game 281
Chapter 16: Dream Big and Visualize Success 285
Chapter 17: The Power of Failure in Running and in Life 289
Chapter 18: Lessons as a Running Coach 293
Chapter 19: World Majors — A Runner's Guide 297

PART 6: RECREATIONAL ATHLETES IN CONVERSATION..........303

Walter Liniger on Joy and Patience......................306
Kofuzi, a.k.a. Mike Ko, on Training Volume......................308
John Birtchet-Sharpe on Self-Acceptance......................310
Astrid Feyer Roberts on Injury Prevention 312
Todd Marentette on Staying Motivated......................314
Eric Floberg on Sub-2:30 Marathons......................316
Jonathan Walton on Success with MAF......................318
Kathryn Geyer on Finding Joy 320
Danny Huibregtse on Enjoyment......................322
Jennifer Kellett on Masters Running 324
Ben Edusei on Training Fundamentals 326
Gareth King on Massive Improvement......................328
Wissam Kheir on Humility......................330
Andy Wheatcroft on Community 332
Josh Sambrook on High Training Volume......................334
Andrea Hudson Baldwin on Visualization......................336
Ash Lewis on His Comeback Story 337
Albert Shank on Ultrarunning......................338
Bill Callahan on Mental Strategies......................339
Larisa Dannis MacFadden on Intuitive Training 340
Nicki Hugie Terry on Body Awareness......................341
Calvin Sambrook on Age Barriers......................342
Greg Nance on Taking the Leap......................343
Jay Motley on Overcoming Barriers 344
Kyle Whalum on Mindful Running......................345
Liam Lonsdale on the Benefits of Trail Running......................346
Martinus Evans on Inclusivity 347
Michael Ovens on Morning Runs......................348
Jessica Dorsey on Mental Strength 349
Kelley Puckett on Racing Strategy 350
Gwen Ostrosky on Breakthroughs......................351
Andy Hooks on the Love of Running......................352

PART 7: GEAR, RESOURCES, AND FINAL INSIGHTS 353

    Chapter 20: Gear Up — Recommendations for Runners 357
    Chapter 21: If You're Feeling Down, Read This 365
    Chapter 22: Lessons from My First 100-Mile (161-km) Run 371

RECOMMENDED RESOURCES 375

TOP 25 EXTRAMILEST PODCASTS 377

FINAL THOUGHTS 379

CONCLUSION: ADVICE TO MY YOUNGER SELF 381

WHAT IT ALL MEANS: THE PRACTICE OF BECOMING 385

NEED EXTRA SUPPORT? 387

ACKNOWLEDGMENTS 391

GLOSSARY 395

START HERE
How to Use This Book

Since my early twenties, I've written down thoughts about my workouts, my races and what I'm learning about running, health and life. These detailed journals captured not just physical metrics but mental breakthroughs, setbacks and everything in between. I found that writing things down helped me see patterns I'd otherwise miss.

Over the past decade, I've also recorded hundreds of conversations with world-class athletes, health and fitness experts, creatives, entrepreneurs and recreational runners. These conversations were often centered around finding ways to become stronger, healthier and happier by optimizing performance in a variety of areas, not just in running but in life.

My approach to these conversations was simple: ask the questions I genuinely wanted answers to. Here are a few questions that consistently yielded the most profound insights:

- Knowing what you know now, what advice would you give to your younger self?
- How can athletes become stronger, healthier and happier?
- How do you handle challenges and setbacks in your training and life?

The answers often surprised me. The world's top performers rarely mentioned secret workouts or miracle supplements. Instead, they spoke about the importance of joy in the process, and about ways to be present, consistent and patient.

Over the years, I've coached more than a thousand runners through my Personal Best Program. What started out as a running podcast quickly became much more, giving me a holistic perspective that transformed how I approach life itself.

Before every podcast, I immerse myself in research: reading my guests' books, studying their interviews, and exploring their philosophies. This is an important part of the process to move beyond standard questions and go deeper than the surface.

I've learned deeply from these teachers. Often, it took listening to the conversations multiple times, slowly digesting their wisdom, to uncover the most valuable insights.

I took detailed notes before, during and after our conversations. More than 20 notebooks, countless pages in Evernote and over 3,000 pages of podcast transcripts later, I had built a personal library of notes and lessons that profoundly shaped my life.

Initially, I never intended to publish these notes. After each podcast episode, I asked our community on YouTube: "What was your favorite lesson, takeaway or quote from this episode?" After more than 20,000 comments, these insights became a powerful, community-driven compilation. Often, listeners highlighted insights that matched mine, but many times, they revealed new perspectives I hadn't noticed. Hearing the profound impact that some podcast episodes have had on people's lives confirmed that I wasn't the only one experiencing positive change.

Recently, on the same day, two people messaged me separately that my podcast and the Personal Best (PB) Program literally saved their life. They were experiencing suicidal thoughts, but they began to feel hope and turned things around to become a happier, healthier and stronger version of themselves. Over the years I've heard hundreds of stories of breakthroughs and transformations from my community. This is one of the reasons why this book is so personal and special to me. It's a calling to get it out in the world and hopefully help more people.

Several podcast guests have become close friends. We've gone on adventures together and collaborated on creative projects. We've shared races around the world, ice baths, long runs, text messages, phone calls and meals together, often trading ideas on what works and what doesn't. These relationships have allowed me to learn and grow far beyond our recorded conversations.

Every training cycle and race experience teaches us something. The small details can absolutely make or break a workout. After running more than 50 races, from distances between 5K and 100 miles, these notes have become invaluable.

I remember, before my first 50-mile (80-km) ultramarathon, I reached out to five experienced ultramarathoners. Nervous about the unknown, I simply asked questions: What advice do you have to someone running their first 50-mile (80-km) race? What common issues have you experienced, and how did you work through these issues?

The more training and racing experience I gained, the more confident I became that everything could be figured out. I'd often reread my notes from previous training cycles and races, and these notes became literal advice for things to keep in mind for my future self, based on past experiences.

Every time I felt stuck, frustrated, uncertain or just needed inspiration, I flipped through these notes. Without fail, within minutes I'd find what I needed: clarity, reassurance, tough love or encouragement. Many valuable insights were hidden deep within thousands of pages of podcast transcripts and handwritten notes.

I had found a rich and detailed source for creating an easily accessible guide, a playbook I could revisit over and over. That was the genesis of this project: something that captured the joys and hardships in running and life and that could be shared to inspire others in their journey.

Writing this book has been a beautiful emotional roller coaster. There were so many golden nuggets that my guests shared over the years, and I couldn't help but tear up on numerous occasions as I revisited these moments, even while writing this introduction. My guests poured their hearts and souls into these conversations, and I tried to do the same with this book.

The first draft ran to more than 700 pages. Through careful editing, I've distilled it down to the essential lessons I wish I'd known when I started this journey. Everything in these pages has been tested, explored and implemented in my own life. I've relied on these strategies on easy training days, during challenging races and through tough times in business and life. These lessons have helped me reach breakthroughs in various areas and saved me years of frustration, providing clarity when it mattered most.

How to Read This Book

This book isn't just a collection of quotes, it's a practical toolkit designed to change your running, your health and your life. Here are some tips on how to get the most out of it.

Skip Around

Feel free to jump from topic to topic rather than reading sequentially. Choose what interests you most. Don't force yourself through anything that doesn't resonate. Enjoyment is key.

I rarely read a book from cover to cover. Each of these chapters can be read on its own, as a standalone chapter.

When skipping sections, though, think about why you're moving past them. Could these skipped topics represent areas of your running or life you've avoided addressing? Sometimes the chapters we resist contain the insights we need most.

Apply Immediately

Knowledge without application is just entertainment. After reading a section that resonates with you, ask yourself: "How can I test this principle in my next run or workout?" Even a small change is better than a big intention. Keep it simple; don't overthink it.

Common Habits for Your Running Success

Throughout the book, you'll notice certain habits and mindsets repeatedly endorsed by the world's best athletes, coaches and recreational runners:

- Everyone experiences challenges. What matters is how you frame your response and work through struggles as part of the journey.
- Enjoying your training and racing is crucial for long-term success beyond race times. Focus on the process, not just the outcome.

- Managing stress and calming the nervous system are key to optimizing your health and performance. Improve your health first and your running performance will follow.
- Meditation and breathwork practices are powerful tools used by many high performers.
- Regular journaling builds self-awareness. Self-kindness, gratitude and patience help build positive momentum.
- Prioritize recovery. Sleep is one of the most underused training tools available.
- Balance consistency in training with flexibility when real-life circumstances happen.
- Continue to learn. Our body and mind evolve over time. Experiment, learn and stay curious.
- Seek flow in your running and life instead of trying to force results.

How This Book Is Structured

This book is organized into clear sections that alternate between practical tools and actionable advice. Look for patterns across chapters and guest insights, and pay attention to recurring themes. These are often the habits and ideas that create lasting change. I've included a glossary of selected terms that might be unfamiliar to readers without an extensive background in running.

About 60% of this book consists of the best questions and answers from my conversations with elite athletes, experts and recreational runners, along with responses from our podcast listeners. About 40% is my own writing from my experiences as a runner, coach, podcast host and dad.

You'll also hear remarkable stories from everyday athletes who've applied the principles from this book to achieve extraordinary breakthroughs. From William Barth, who rediscovered his running potential at 70, to Duc Tran, who finally broke the sub-3-hour marathon barrier, these case studies show what's possible when you embrace a smarter, more holistic approach.

As I said earlier, over the years, I've coached more than a thousand runners, and most of them are their own harshest critics. When we practice kindness and gratitude toward ourselves, slow down and reduce the pressure, frustration often transforms into profound joy and lasting improvements. Running becomes a source of calm, clarity and happiness.

This book isn't about quick fixes but rather playing the long game, planning strategically, overcoming challenges patiently and making wise decisions consistently. My hope is that this book will support you in all these areas.

I wrote this book to offer practical tools and ideas that have truly worked for me and others. My wish is that you'll find inspiration and guidance within these pages to elevate your running, health and life.

Much love,
Floris Gierman
Irvine, California

/ PART 1

Foundations

Running shouldn't feel like a constant struggle. Yet for many of us, that's exactly how it starts: pushing hard on every run, fighting for breath, dealing with injuries and wondering why we're not getting faster despite all the effort. I've heard this repeatedly, and this was my story, too. For years, I thought the only way to improve was to push harder, run faster and ignore the signals my body was sending me.

That approach left me frustrated, exhausted and frequently injured. Then everything changed. I discovered a smarter way to train that allowed me to run with more joy, and become a stronger and healthier runner. Ultimately, it has helped me to run more than 17,000 miles (27,000 km) over the past decade, complete the World Marathon Majors and take on ultramarathons from 50K to 100 miles. I've also logged personal best times of 1:19 in the half-marathon, 2:44 in the marathon, 50K (31 miles) in 3:30, 50 miles (80 km) in 6:42 and 100 miles (161 km) in 17:47.

I went from not knowing much about running to feeling in control, knowing exactly what to do and why, running in a flow state and completely enjoying the process.

Part 1 of this book lays out the essential building blocks that transformed my running and the running lives of athletes I've worked with through our Personal Best Program. You'll learn why training at a healthy heart rate can actually make you faster and move with more efficiency and ease, as well as how to build a strong aerobic foundation to prevent injuries.

These aren't just theories. They're proven principles backed by exercise science and real-world results. The chapters ahead will help you break through plateaus, reduce injuries and enjoy your running more than ever, whether you're just starting out or have been running for years.

This is the information I wish I'd had when I first started running. It would have saved me years of frustration, injuries and setbacks. My hope is that by understanding these core principles, you can avoid the common pitfalls that hold many runners back and instead build a strong foundation for long-term success and enjoyment in your running journey.

1
How to Run Longer Without Running Out of Breath

I remember standing at the convention center in Long Beach, California. I'd been pushing myself through another grueling training run. It struck me, as it had many times since I'd started training in 2007, that I really didn't like running all that much. The constant struggle to work harder left my legs burning, my sides cramping and my lungs gasping for air. That was what I thought I needed to do to become a better runner.

If you've ever felt this way, you're not alone. Many runners struggle with similar challenges. Here's what I've discovered since that day in Long Beach: Running out of breath isn't a sign that you'll never be a successful runner. It just means that you're running too hard for your current fitness level.

Why You Get Winded (and How to Fix It)

When you run out of breath, your body is desperately trying to get more oxygen to your muscles. Think of it like revving a car engine into the red zone. It's unsustainable, and you'll eventually be forced to slow down or stop.

Here's what's happening inside your body:

- Your muscles need more oxygen than your heart and lungs can deliver
- You slip into a state of anaerobic metabolism (working without enough oxygen)
- Lactic acid builds up, making your muscles burn
- Your breathing becomes rapid and shallow as your body panics for more air

The solution isn't to push through the discomfort. The solution is to slow down.

> **KEEP IN MIND:** "Easy" varies. If you can't chat comfortably, slow down, even to walking or run/walk intervals. Low-intensity training builds the foundation that allows harder efforts when they matter.

In my early years of running, I experienced all the physical discomfort, injury, overtraining, burnout, mental frustration and self-doubt. Then one day, everything changed.

Slow Down to Speed Up

In 2013, I heard Dr. Phil Maffetone on a podcast talking about low heart rate training. It required slowing my pace to where I could maintain a heart rate low enough to carry on a conversation while running.

When I first tried low heart rate training, my ego took a big hit. I set an alarm for a specific heart rate and almost immediately had to slow my pace. I even had to walk, at times, while older runners zipped past me, and I just kept thinking, "This is so frustrating! Is this really going to make me faster? I can't be doing this right!?" Trust me, many of us have had similar thoughts, early on, with low heart rate training.

But after about four weeks of consistent easy running, something incredible happened: My pace at the same heart rate improved by 38 seconds per mile (24 seconds per km). The runs that once felt agonizingly slow were now significantly faster.

> **TRY THIS:** Set out to run at a pace where you could comfortably chat with a friend for the entire duration. Don't worry about your watch or monitor. Focus only on your breathing.

Building Your Body's Engine

Think of your aerobic system as your body's engine for endurance. By running at easy, conversational intensities, your body makes several powerful adaptations:

- **Your Heart Gets Stronger:** It pumps more blood with each beat, delivering oxygen more efficiently.
- **Your Muscles Grow More "Delivery Trucks":** You develop more capillaries (tiny blood vessels that deliver oxygen to working muscles).
- **Your Cells Build More "Power Plants":** You produce more mitochondria, the cellular structures that turn oxygen into energy.
- **You Become a Better Fat Burner:** Fat provides more than twice the energy per gram compared to carbohydrates. Training at low intensity teaches your body to use this abundant fuel source efficiently.

This approach builds a stronger, more efficient aerobic system, ultimately allowing you to run faster and farther when it matters most.

Useful Breathing Techniques

Aside from slowing your pace, these breathing techniques can help you run longer with greater comfort:

The Talk Test

Say something out loud occasionally, while running. If you can speak a complete sentence without gasping, you're in the right zone. If you can't, then slow down.

Breathe Through Your Nose

Try breathing only through your nose during easy runs. This naturally regulates your pace and improves breathing efficiency. If you need to open your mouth to breathe, you're working too hard.

Belly Breathing

Instead of shallow chest breathing, breathe deeply so your belly expands. This draws air deep into your lungs and has a calming effect on your nervous system.

Find Your Rhythm

Try breathing in a rhythm with your steps. A common pattern for easy running is 3:3. Inhale for three steps, then exhale for the next three. Experiment to find what feels natural for you.

From Struggle to Joy

After training at a lower heart rate, I was running faster at a lower intensity, and with less effort. I saw clear proof that my running form had become more relaxed, and the frequent injuries I used to experience had faded away. I could train consistently without long recovery periods.

Most surprisingly, I found joy in running again. It became meditative when I stopped pushing myself to the breaking point. I began looking forward to my runs instead of dreading them.

Putting low-intensity running at the core of my training improved my performance and renewed my love for the sport. I finished my runs feeling energized instead of defeated. Running now gave me time to clear my head, to increase my energy levels and to build fitness without suffering.

> **REMEMBER:** Most of your runs should leave you feeling energized, not depleted. If you finish thinking, "I could do that again," you've nailed it.

The Big Picture

Low heart rate training has changed my life. It could change yours. Don't take my word for it. Just give yourself permission to slow down your running pace or take walk breaks if needed. Ditch the ego and trust the process. Patience is key. Improvements won't happen overnight, but they will come. A whole new level of joy in running awaits!

Running mostly at low intensity transformed both my performance and my mindset. It made me more present and in tune with my body. It's about balance, enjoying the process, staying consistent and understanding that progress happens over time.

Whether you're a seasoned runner or are just starting, remember that sometimes the best way to get faster is to embrace going slower. You'll be amazed at how much farther you can go (and happier you can be) when you stop racing yourself every day and learn to slow down to speed up.

6 Months' Progression

Here's what this type of progress can look like over a longer timeframe. James, a 45-year-old runner, tracked his pace at a heart rate of 135 beats per minute for 6 months.

Changes in Pace over a 6-Month Period at a Heart Rate of 135 Beats per Minute

MONTH	ZONE 2 (MIN/MILE)	ZONE 2 (MIN/KM)
MONTH 1	11:30 MIN / MILE	7:09 MIN / KM
MONTH 2	11:28 MIN / MILE	7:08 MIN / KM
MONTH 3	11:10 MIN / MILE	6:56 MIN / KM
MONTH 4	11:00 MIN / MILE	6:50 MIN / KM
MONTH 5	10:55 MIN / MILE	6:47 MIN / KM
MONTH 6	10:32 MIN / MILE	6:33 MIN / KM

I have personally experienced similar results, improving at the same low heart rate by 2 minutes and 10 seconds per mile (1:21 per km) over an 18-month period.

Chapter Summary

- **Slow Down to Speed Up:** Running out of breath means you're pushing too hard for your current fitness; reduce your pace to conversational effort to effectively build aerobic endurance.
- **Optimize Your Breathing:** Use practical breathing methods, like the talk test, nasal breathing and rhythmic breathing. This maintains optimal intensity, improves running efficiency and increases comfort.
- **Discover the Joy of Running:** Embracing low heart rate training transforms running into a more relaxed, injury-free and enjoyable practice, enabling sustainable and measurable progress.

2
Start (or Restart) Your Running Journey

Training can feel harder than it should for runners at every experience level. Building fitness, or rebuilding after an injury or long break, presents universal challenges. This chapter discusses proven strategies for creating a solid foundation for fitness without unnecessary struggle so you can move forward confidently in your practice.

Start Where You Are

I made an all-too-common mistake when I began running. I tried to do too much too soon. After years of struggle, I finally learned the importance of starting where I was, not where I thought I should be. This simple shift in mindset applies whether you're a complete beginner or an experienced runner returning from a break, injury or burnout.

It's a lesson that I must keep learning. At peak fitness, a 2-hour run at a solid pace feels almost effortless to me. Time flies by, and my body moves with confidence and energy. But when I return from an injury or a pause in training, or when I begin a new cycle, even a short jog can feel like an eternity. It's a powerful reminder that fitness isn't permanent and requires consistent cultivation.

The key to my success was embracing my current fitness reality without judgment. If you can only run 30 seconds before needing to walk, that's your perfect starting point. If you're an experienced runner coming back from a break, your pace and endurance today, not six months ago, is your foundation.

Resist the urge to compare yourself to a previous peak fitness level. I've been there, and that mindset does more harm than good.

A Progressive Training Framework for All Levels

If you're just starting out:

- Begin with three 20-minute sessions per week
- Start with a 5-minute walk
- Then use run/walk intervals (1 minute running, 1 minute walking)
- Gradually extend running-interval duration as comfort improves
- Try to maintain an easy, conversational effort, and take walk breaks whenever needed

If you're returning from an injury or a break:

- Reduce your previous typical training volume (either in time or distance) by 50%–70%
- Prioritize frequency (three to five short time-based runs) over aiming for longer distance
- Keep your runs at an easy pace
- Increase volume by no more than 10% weekly, and take a step back of 30%–40% less volume every fourth week

Base Building for Recovery

After intense training blocks, half-marathons or marathons, implement a deliberate two- or three-week "aerobic reset" where you:

- Eliminate all high-intensity work
- Focus exclusively on enjoyment and form
- Run by feel instead of following a strict schedule
- Gradually rebuild volume at an easy pace

Even Olympic athletes regularly return to base-building periods focused on easy running. These aren't steps backward but rather strategic resets that enable new levels of performance by:

- Re-establishing aerobic efficiency
- Healing subtle overuse issues before they become injuries
- Renewing mental freshness and motivation
- Building new capillary networks to support harder future training

High-intensity training creates micro-tears in your muscles, which is a normal part of building strength. Pushing too hard too soon after a race can lead to injury if these micro-tears haven't healed.

By adding recovery periods into your annual training plan, you create the foundation for future breakthroughs while preventing burnout and injuries. This isn't a step backward. It sets the stage for even greater achievements in the future.

The Time-on-Feet Approach

Using the metric of the time you spend moving, rather than pace or the distance you cover, is an excellent method for keeping your focus on where you are. It removes unnecessary pressure and helps you tune in to how your body feels. You know instinctively what 20 or 60 minutes is, regardless of the pace. I've seen this play out many times. The two examples below illustrate this well.

Anna is a beginning runner and member of our Personal Best Program. She started with short 30-second runs between walk breaks. Four months later, she finished her first 5K. How? She showed up consistently for three weekly training sessions without judging herself for needing walk breaks.

James, an experienced marathoner, broke through years of plateaus and injuries by running for six months, mostly at an easy conversational pace, and with only a handful of speed sessions. The result? He had his first injury-free year in nearly a decade and shaved 17 minutes off his marathon personal record (PR).

Managing Common Challenges

The Comparison Trap: Whether you're comparing yourself to others or to your former self, this mindset only leads to frustration. Focus instead on consistent progress from where you are today.

Impatience: The body adapts at its own pace. Beginners often expect dramatic weekly improvements, while returning runners get frustrated when they can't immediately hit their previous paces. Trust the gradual process of adaptation.

The Identity Challenge: Many experienced runners struggle with ego when returning from a break, feeling as though they've "lost" their running identity. Remember that accepting your current fitness and rebuilding patiently demonstrates greater athletic maturity than pushing too hard too soon.

Patience and Commitment Are the True Keys to Success

Whether you're taking your first running steps or your millionth, celebrate your commitment to the process. Success isn't measured by speed or distance alone, but by your consistency and patience.

- Did you show up today? That's a win.
- Did you respect your body's feedback? Another win.
- Are you building sustainability into your running? That's the ultimate win.
- Did you find a way to enjoy your run? That's what matters most to me.

Remember to start where you are today, run at a pace that feels right for your current fitness level, build up slowly and keep showing up.

You've already got past the hardest part by deciding to start your running journey. So keep moving forward at a pace that feels right for where you are now. It will transform your running just as it has mine.

Chapter Summary

- **Accept Your Starting Point:** Begin training at your current fitness level, without judgment or comparison, to establish a realistic, injury-free foundation for long-term improvement.
- **Build Progressively and Sustainably:** Focus on short, frequent sessions at an easy conversational pace. Gradually increase training volume by around 10% per week to avoid burnout and enhance consistency.
- **Prioritize Time over Pace:** Use time on feet rather than speed or distance to reduce pressure, foster body awareness and consistently celebrate your commitment to the running journey.

3
Heart Rate Training Fundamentals

Every runner has a personal compass that guides both their immediate performance and their long-term development. This compass is your heart rate.

When I first began training by heart rate, I felt lost in a sea of confusing numbers and formulas. Should I use 220 minus my age? What about the MAF 180 Formula? These questions plagued me until I tested different approaches and discovered what worked best for my body.

> **TRY THIS:** On your next run, check two simple indicators: Can you speak in complete sentences without gasping? Can you comfortably breathe through your nose? If you answer yes to both, you're likely in the right aerobic zone. If not, simply slow down.

The 80/20 Principle: Nature's Training Balance

Dr. Stephen Seiler, an exercise physiologist, appeared on my Extramilest podcast (Ep. 50) and shared what he considers the key to long-term athletic success: training intensity distribution. His research revealed a fascinating pattern among elite endurance athletes across different sports:

Most of the successful elite endurance athletes train at comfortable intensities about 80% of the time, in some cases 90% of the time.

This isn't just a preference but a pattern that emerges naturally when athletes listen to their bodies over time. Like many patterns in nature, this balance seems to optimize both stress and recovery for long-term development.

For many elite athletes, most of that easy work is Zone 1, not Zone 2.

Why are there benefits to training in Zone 1 instead of Zone 2, especially if you train at a higher volume? Because consistency trumps intensity. Zone 1 allows you to:

- Accumulate more volume without fatigue
- Recover fully between harder sessions
- Build sustainable habits over months and years

For elite athletes, the remaining 10%–20% includes strategic harder sessions that vary across all intensities. That's not just maximum effort, but everything in between. All zones matter at different times.

The Middle Zone Trap

Most runners get stuck in the no man's land of medium intensity, where they work too hard to build proper aerobic fitness but not hard enough to produce maximum speed gains. It feels productive in the moment but undermines long-term progress.

WHAT MANY RECREATIONAL RUNNERS DO

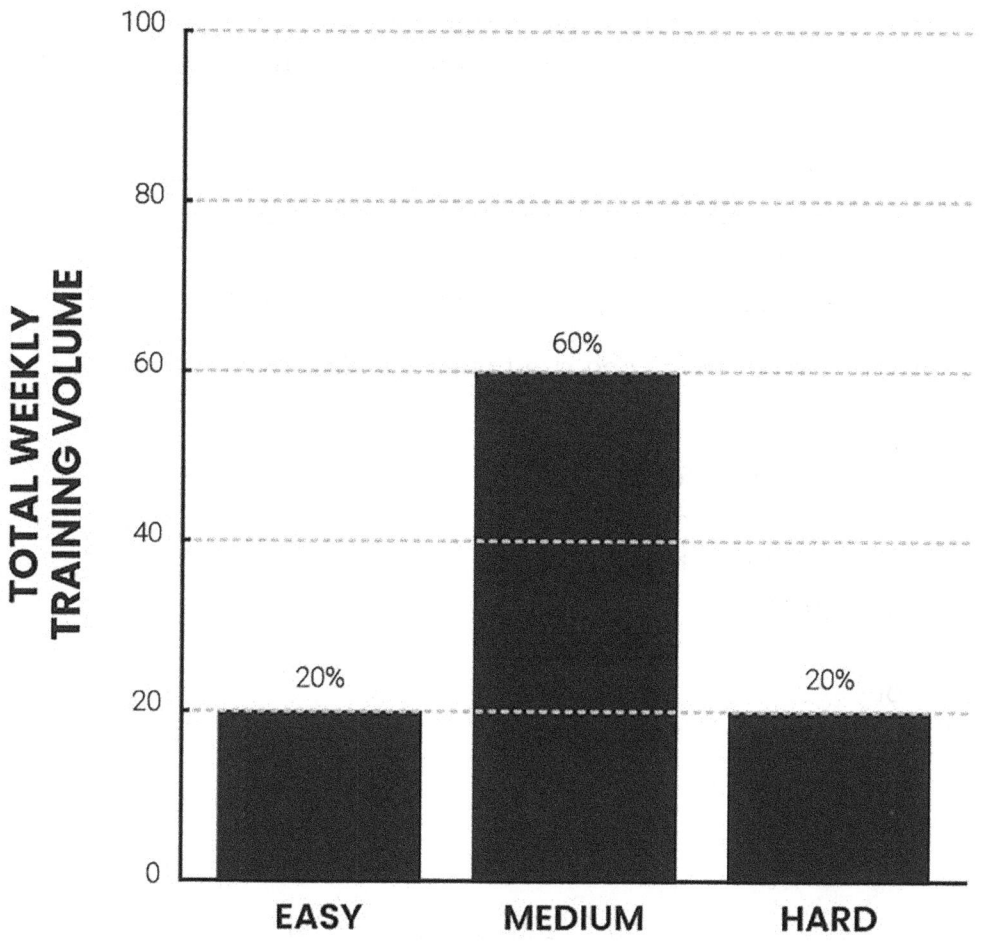

KEEP IN MIND: If your runs always feel "kinda hard," you're stuck in the middle zone. Slow down significantly for easy days, or deliberately push harder for targeted workouts. All zones have their place; the key is being intentional about which one you're using.

Beyond "Low" or "High": Healthy Heart Rate Training

In my conversation with movement specialist Lawrence van Lingen, we discussed *healthy* heart rate training instead of low heart rate or high heart rate training. The distinction might seem small, but it makes a world of difference.

Maintaining a healthy heart rate during training isn't always about keeping it low but ensuring that you're flexible and training smart. It's about recognizing when your body needs:

- Less effort to build your aerobic base, meaning your body gets better at running longer without getting tired as quickly
- Less effort to recover properly
- More effort to mix things up and sharpen your fitness

Heart rate training is not one-size-fits-all. Your ideal training zones depend on several factors, such as:

- Your training history
- Your current overall fitness
- Your health profile and potential injuries
- Your stress levels
- Your available time to train
- Your age
- Your natural physiology
- Your race goals
- The weather
- The altitude

The objective is to train consistently and improve with joy, without breaking down your body and mind.

Case Study
Daniel Edwards: Finding Joy in Sustainable Running at 51

Daniel Edwards has been running, on and off, since 2016. Despite completing four marathons, he felt none had gone according to plan.

"I didn't stand a chance at being successful," Daniel said. "All I was doing was running and trying to run harder. I stayed sore the whole time. It wasn't sustainable for any period."

At almost 50 years old and recovering from neck surgery, Daniel was searching for a healthier approach. After seeing his friend Greg's dramatic improvement using low heart rate training, Daniel decided to give our Personal Best Program a try.

Two years later, the results speak for themselves. At 51, Daniel is in the best shape of his life, setting personal records in every distance from 5K to marathon. At the Richmond Marathon, he shattered his previous year's time by over 30 minutes, finishing in 3:43.

The Transformation: Training Smarter, Not Harder

The transition to low heart rate training wasn't easy for Daniel. Like many runners new to the method, he was humbled by how slow he needed to run, to stay in Zone 2.

"It's a tough pill to swallow when you go out trying to run in Zone 2 and you can't without having to walk," he says. "You think, 'I thought I was in better shape than this.'"

But Daniel trusted the process despite the initial challenges. What kept him motivated was how much easier the training felt compared to his previous approach.

"It doesn't even really seem fair because it's so much easier than what I was doing before. When you can do something that is much easier and get a better result, that's just a no-brainer."

This sustainability was key for Daniel: "I was looking for something I could continue to do when I'm 71 or 81, something that would age with me. A lot of training programs are just too intense to maintain as you age."

Beyond Running: A Holistic Approach

Daniel's success comes from more than just changing his running style. He embraced a comprehensive approach:

> **Daily Strength Work:** Daniel performs a 19-minute core routine every morning, completing 15 1-minute exercises. "It's just part of my routine now, like brushing my teeth."
>
> **Nutrition Transformation:** Working with a dietician, Daniel optimized his diet. "I feel a lot better when I don't eat poison."
>
> **Race-Fueling Strategy:** As someone with type 1 diabetes, Daniel carefully manages his nutrition during races. "I set a timer on my watch to take a gel every 30 minutes. If your blood sugar gets low during a race, it's really hard to recover."

Rediscovering Joy in Running

Perhaps the most significant change was how Daniel approached races. Instead of treating every event as a do-or-die effort, he learned to enjoy the experience.

"This year, my training partner Greg and I did races where we didn't have any goals. We went to the Cooper River Bridge Run and ran up the bridge backwards, taking pictures. We had an awesome time."

This new mindset paid off during his breakthrough Richmond Marathon. "My training showed up regardless of how I felt. I wasn't having to use a lot of grit. My body was doing what we trained it to do. I've been smiling ever since."

Daniel also developed a healthier relationship with running itself. "Running makes me happy, but it doesn't control my happiness. If I couldn't run anymore, I'd still need to find a way to be happy."

The Road Ahead

At 51, Daniel is running better than he did in his forties. With his training dialed in, he and Greg have set an ambitious goal: to qualify for the Boston Marathon within the next five years.

For newer runners, Daniel offers straightforward advice: "Do your research. If you're looking to change your lifestyle and do something sustainable, give this approach a try."

Daniel's transformation proves that with the right approach to training, nutrition and recovery, reaching your potential as a runner is possible at any age, and you can enjoy the journey along the way.

Full Episode:
extramilest.com/94

The Science Behind the Zones

> *The better your cardiorespiratory fitness, the better your brain works: better executive function, better memory, better processing speed.*
> —Dr. Andrew Huberman

Dr. Peter Attia, a physician and former endurance athlete, has identified Zone 2 (where the body produces lactic acid at a rate of less than 2 millimoles per liter) as the sweet spot for health and endurance development.

For now, it's important to note that Zone 2 is where you challenge your aerobic system without shifting significantly into anaerobic energy production. Think of it as the "Goldilocks zone": It's not too easy, and not too hard, but just right.

Understanding the Training Zones

Before diving into detailed calculation methods in the next chapter, let's look at what each training zone represents:

Zone 1: Recovery

- **Feel:** Very easy, could maintain all day
- **Talking:** Full conversations with no effort
- **Purpose:** Active recovery, warm-ups, cooldowns, building aerobic capacity
- **When to use:** After hard workouts, when fatigued, when easing back from injury, during high training-load weeks

Zone 2: Aerobic Development

- **Feel:** Comfortable but purposeful
- **Talking:** Complete sentences, slightly elevated breathing
- **Purpose:** Building aerobic capacity and fat-burning efficiency
- **When to use:** Most regular runs, long runs

Zone 3: Tempo

- **Feel:** "Comfortably hard," sustained effort
- **Talking:** Short phrases between breaths
- **Purpose:** Builds endurance and lactate clearance
- **When to use:** Tempo runs, sustained efforts

Zone 4: Threshold

- **Feel:** Hard but sustainable for limited time
- **Talking:** Only a few words at a time
- **Purpose:** Improves lactate threshold (the point where your muscles start to burn) and race-specific fitness
- **When to use:** Interval workouts, race preparation

Zone 5: Maximum

- **Feel:** Near-maximum effort, hard to sustain
- **Talking:** Usually not possible beyond a word or two
- **Purpose:** Improves power, speed and VO_2 max
- **When to use:** Short intervals, final race preparation (with caution)

> **REMEMBER:** Most athletes will benefit from 80%–90% of their training in Zones 1–2. If you're always in Zones 3–4, you're making running harder than it needs to be.

Special Focus: Base Building

For runners returning from injury, recovering from burnout, building a foundation or hitting a plateau, there can be tremendous value in spending a defined period (usually 8 to 12 weeks) focused exclusively on Zone 1–2 training.

This approach is especially powerful for athletes whose race times have stagnated despite increasing training volume or intensity. Think of it like trying to build a skyscraper on a foundation designed for a small house.

Exclusive low-intensity training:

- Allows tissues to strengthen gradually
- Builds cardiovascular efficiency with less strain
- Develops fat-burning metabolic pathways
- Resets the nervous system after periods of high stress
- Corrects muscular imbalances that limit performance
- Creates a foundation for more effective high-intensity training later

Sara's Breakthrough: Sara had been stuck at the same half-marathon time for three years despite adding more speed work. After 10 weeks of exclusive low-intensity training in Zones 1 and 2, her easy pace improved by over a minute per mile (37 sec/km) at the same heart rate. When she reintroduced intensity, she broke her half-marathon personal best by 7 minutes.

> **REMEMBER:** Don't make the mistake of thinking that easy training won't make you faster. The biggest improvements often come from building a stronger foundation, not adding more intensity to a weak base.

Next Steps

Take a moment to consider your current running:

1. In the past month, what percentage of your running has been easy enough for you to hold a conversation?
2. Do you often finish runs feeling depleted or energized?
3. If someone asked you to go for another run later the same day you'd already been out, would that seem possible most days?

If less than 80% of your running is at a conversational pace, or if you regularly finish runs feeling depleted, you might benefit from adjusting your training intensity distribution.

Chapter Summary

- Most successful endurance athletes train about 80%–90% of their time at low intensity and 10%–20% at moderate to high intensity.
- Heart rate training can provide a personal "compass" to ensure you're training at the right intensity.
- Finding your optimal training zones is the first step toward more enjoyable, sustainable and effective running.

In the next chapter, we'll explore practical methods to calculate your personal heart rate zones so you can train with precision and purpose.

4
Calculating Your Personal Heart Rate Zones

The greatest performance gains come from the first approximation of doing things right versus doing them wrong. It's not about fancy interval protocols or high-tech equipment. It's about getting the fundamentals of training intensity distribution right.

—Dr. Stephen Seiler

Finding Your Optimal Training Intensity

Now that you understand why training at the right intensity is critical, let's explore how to find your optimal heart rate zones. Think of this chapter as your personal heart rate laboratory.

We'll start with the simplest methods that require no equipment and progressively move toward more precise approaches. For each method, I'll share:

- Quick start
- Who it works best for
- A real-world example
- Troubleshooting tips
- The pros and cons

> **REMEMBER:** There's no single "perfect" method. By the end of this chapter, you'll understand which method (or combination) works best for your unique situation.

Method 1: The Talk Test

Quick Start: During your run, try having a conversation with a running partner or speaking on the phone. If you can do this comfortably, you're in the right zone for aerobic development.

The talk test is the simplest way to identify different intensity zones using only your breathing:

- **Zones 1–2 (Easy/Aerobic):** Complete sentences flow easily
- **Zone 3 (Moderate):** Short phrases between breaths
- **Zones 4–5 (Hard):** Only a few words at a time, or no talking possible

Who It's Best For

- Beginners just starting with intensity management
- Runners who don't have or don't want to use heart rate monitors
- Athletes who train in environments where heart rate can be misleading (extreme heat or cold, altitude, etc.)
- Anyone looking for a free, intuitive method

A Real-World Example: John's Experience

John, a 45-year-old new runner, found himself constantly exhausted after runs. When he joined our training group, I asked him to maintain a pace where he could comfortably chat with a friend.

Initially, this meant slowing to what felt like a crawl, even incorporating walking breaks. Three months later, he completed his first 10K at a pace that previously would have left him breathless, all while maintaining conversation with his running partner.

Troubleshooting Tips: The Talk Test

Challenge	Solution
"I feel too slow when I can talk easily"	Remember, this is temporary; your talking pace will get faster as fitness improves
"I can talk at the start but not later in the run"	This is normal cardiac drift; slow down as needed to maintain talking ability
"I feel awkward talking during runs"	Try counting to 10 aloud instead, or recite a familiar phrase
"My breathing seems fine, but my legs are burning"	This indicates local muscle fatigue; build more base mileage at this easy pace

Advantages

- Requires no equipment
- Works anywhere, anytime
- Accounts for daily fluctuations in your physical state
- Automatically adjusts to environmental conditions (heat, humidity, etc.)

Limitations

- Less precise for intentional zone transitions
- Perception of "conversational pace" varies between individuals
- More difficult to use for interval training with quick intensity changes

TRY THIS: Have an actual phone conversation with a friend during your run. If you find yourself breathing hard or struggling to speak, slow down until conversation flows naturally.

Method 2: Nose Breathing

Quick Start: On your next run, breathe only through your nose. When you start to feel the need to open your mouth to breathe, you've left your aerobic zone.

Nose breathing naturally limits your intensity and helps identify your zones:

- **Zones 1–2 (Easy/Aerobic):** Comfortable breathing through nose only
- **Zone 3 (Moderate):** Nasal breathing becomes challenging
- **Zones 4–5 (Hard):** Need to breathe through mouth

Dr. Andrew Huberman notes, in an episode of his podcast, that nasal breathing is "a reliable indicator of aerobic intensity, naturally guiding you into the right training zone." Breathing patterns respond more quickly to intensity changes than heart rate, offering immediate, intuitive feedback.

Who It's Best For

- Runners looking to develop better breathing efficiency
- Those who tend to push too hard during easy runs
- Runners looking to train without technology
- Athletes with inconsistent heart rate responses
- Individuals prone to exercise-induced asthma (nasal breathing warms and filters air)

A Real-World Example: Mia's Transformation

Mia was a "Type A" runner who constantly pushed herself into the high-intensity zone on every run. Despite increasing her training volume, her half-marathon times stagnated at 1:55 for three years.

When she committed to nose-breathing runs for 8 weeks, she initially had to slow her pace by nearly 2 minutes per mile (1:15 per km). By week 8, she could maintain her previous "normal" pace while breathing mostly through her nose. A month later, she ran a 1:47 half-marathon with less perceived effort than her previous races, an 8-minute personal best.

Troubleshooting Tips: Nose Breathing

Challenge	Solution
"My nose starts dripping (runny) during runs"	This is normal during the initial weeks of nasal breathing on your runs
"Hills make nasal breathing impossible"	Either slow down significantly on hills or take walking breaks while maintaining nose breathing
"I feel like I'm not getting enough air"	Slow your pace more; try nasal strips to open your nostrils; start with short intervals of nose breathing

Advantages

- No equipment needed (unless using nasal strips)
- Creates a natural "limiter" preventing overexertion
- Improves breathing efficiency over time
- Provides immediate feedback on intensity

Limitations

- Not precise for determining exact heart rate zones
- Individual differences in nasal passage size affect results
- Can be challenging with allergies or congestion
- As efficiency improves, your zones can change

Method 3: The MAF Method (180 Formula)

Quick Start: Subtract your age from 180 to find your maximum aerobic heart rate. Stay at or below this number during all aerobic training sessions.

The MAF Method, developed by Dr. Phil Maffetone, uses a simple formula to find your aerobic heart rate:

1. **Start with 180 minus your age** to get your base MAF number
2. **Adjust based on your current health and fitness:**
   - **Subtract 10** if you have a major illness, regularly take medication, are recovering from surgery or suffer chronic overtraining
   - **Subtract 5** if you have infections, allergies, asthma, injuries, aren't improving, have excess body fat or are new to training
   - **No adjustment** if you've trained consistently (4+ times per week) for up to two years without issues
   - **Add 5** if you've trained consistently over two years and remain injury-free
3. Your MAF zone ranges from 10 beats below your MAF number up to your MAF number

Example: For a healthy 40-year-old runner, 180 − 40 = 140 bpm. So, MAF zone = 130–140 bpm.

Who It's Best For

- Runners returning from injury
- Those who tend to overtrain
- Anyone building an aerobic base
- Athletes who have hit performance plateaus
- Runners with a history of injury or burnout
- Competitive runners looking to strengthen their foundation

A Real-World Example: Michael's Comeback

Michael, a 38-year-old marathoner, had completed six marathons at around 3:45 but developed persistent knee pain. After his last race, he developed persistent knee pain that wouldn't resolve despite six months of physical therapy. When he joined our training program, we calculated his MAF rate at 137 bpm (180 − 38 − 5).

His initial pace at this heart rate was nearly 12 minutes per mile (7:27 min/km), a shock for someone used to training at 8:30 min/mile pace (5:17 min/km). After 12 weeks of strict MAF training, his pace at 137 bpm improved to 9:45/mile (6:04/km). More importantly, he trained pain-free.

Three months later, his MAF pace dropped to 9:05/mile (5:39/km). He then ran a 3:29 marathon with negative splits and no knee pain, despite significantly less weekly mileage than his previous training cycles.

Troubleshooting Tips: The MAF Method

Challenge	Solution
"My MAF pace is embarrassingly slow"	Everyone starts somewhere; focus on the process, not the current pace
"My heart rate spikes too quickly"	Start with run/walk intervals (run until HR reaches MAF; walk until it drops to MAF-10)
"I can't keep my heart rate low enough on any incline"	Walk all hills initially; your ability to run inclines while maintaining MAF will improve
"My MAF pace isn't improving after several weeks/months"	Check recovery factors (sleep, nutrition, stress); make sure you train enough, for at least 4 or 5 hours/week aerobically; ensure you're truly staying at or below MAF

Advantages

- Simple to calculate and remember
- Takes health and fitness into account
- No maximum heart rate test needed
- Automatically adjusts as you age
- Has helped thousands improve performance while reducing injuries

Limitations

- Less accurate for individuals with unusually high/low maximum heart rates
- May need further personalization for athletes over 55
- Can lead to extremely slow running or walking initially, which some find discouraging
- Requires honest self-assessment for proper category selection

> **REMEMBER:** The MAF Method forces you to build a foundation before adding intensity. Trust the process even when it feels slow.

Method 4: Zone Training: Percentage of Maximum Heart Rate

Quick Start: Estimate your maximum heart rate with 220 minus your age. Multiply by 0.60 and 0.70 to find your Zone 2 range.

Example: A 40-year-old would have an estimated max HR of 180, making their Zone 2 range 108–126 bpm.

This method estimates training zones based on percentages of maximum heart rate:

1. Determine your maximum heart rate through either:
   - **Estimation formula:** 220 minus your age (though this can be inaccurate)
   - **Field test:** structured workout approaching maximum effort
2. Calculate zones based on percentages:
   - **Zone 1 (Very Easy):** 50%–60% of max HR
   - **Zone 2 (Easy/Aerobic):** 60%–70% of max HR
   - **Zone 3 (Moderate):** 70%–80% of max HR
   - **Zone 4 (Threshold):** 80%–90% of max HR
   - **Zone 5 (Maximum):** 90%–100% of max HR

Field Test Protocol to Determine Your Max Heart Rate

After a thorough warm-up, perform 3–4 progressive all-out efforts of 2–3 minutes each, with recovery between. Adding a hill can help. Note your highest heart rate, understanding that this may still be below your true maximum.

Who It's Best For

- Runners enjoying structured training with different intensities
- Athletes who have accurately determined their true maximum heart rate

A Real-World Example: Samantha's Structured Approach

Samantha, a 32-year-old recreational runner, struggled with inconsistent training and didn't know how fast to run. After determining her max heart rate was 192 through a field test (higher than the age-predicted 188), she established clear zones.

She assigned specific purposes to each run: recovery runs in Zone 1 (96–115 bpm); base building in Zone 2 (115–134 bpm); tempo in Zone 3 (134–154 bpm) and intervals in Zone 4 (154–173 bpm).

Over 6 months, she improved her 5K time from 26:38 to 23:15, while enjoying her training more than ever.

Troubleshooting Tips: Percentage-Based Zones

Challenge	Solution
"My estimated max heart rate doesn't seem accurate"	Consider a field test, or adjust zones based on perceived effort
"I find it difficult to stay in the assigned zones"	Create buffer zones of ±2–3 beats; focus on the purpose of the run rather than exact numbers
"My zones feel too low/high compared to my perceived effort"	Your max HR may differ from age-predicted formulas; adjust based on your field max HR test results
"I'm afraid to do a max HR test"	Use a submaximal test (like 20 minutes at hard effort) and add 5–10 beats to your highest reading

Advantages

- Creates ranges rather than a single number
- 220-minus-age formula scales with age
- Widely understood in training programs
- Provides clear zones for different training purposes

Limitations

- The 220-minus-age formula is often inaccurate
- Field tests carry injury risk
- Many don't push hard enough during tests to reach true maximum
- Doesn't account for individual variations in heart rate response

Method 5: Heart Rate Reserve Method (Karvonen Formula)

Quick Start: Measure your resting heart rate first thing in the morning. Subtract this from your maximum heart rate to find your "heart rate reserve." Calculate percentages of this reserve, then add back your resting heart rate.

The Heart Rate Reserve Method offers a more personalized approach:

1. **Measure your resting heart rate** first thing in the morning before getting out of bed
2. **Measure or estimate your maximum heart** rate (220 minus age)
3. **Calculate your heart rate reserve (HRR):** Maximum HR minus resting HR
4. **Determine your zones using percentages of your HRR, then add your resting HR:**
   - **Zone 1:** 50%–60% of HRR + resting HR
   - **Zone 2:** 60%–70% of HRR + resting HR
   - **Zone 3:** 70%–80% of HRR + resting HR
   - **Zone 4:** 80%–90% of HRR + resting HR
   - **Zone 5:** 90%–100% of HRR + resting HR

Who It's Best For

- Runners seeking greater precision
- Those with accurate maximum and resting heart rate values
- Athletes whose fitness is changing rapidly
- Runners with unusually high or low resting heart rates

A Real-World Example: David's Personalization Journey

David, a 51-year-old runner with 15 years of experience, found standard heart rate formulas frustrating. With a resting heart rate of 42 bpm and measured maximum of 195 bpm (higher than age-predicted), standard formulas put him in zones that felt wrong.

Using heart rate reserve, his Zone 2 calculated to 134–149 bpm (vs. 117–136 using simple percentages). This personalized range aligned well with his talk test results and subjective effort. With newly calibrated zones, David successfully completed his first 50K race.

Troubleshooting Tips: Heart Rate Reserve Method

Challenge	Solution
"The calculations seem complicated"	Use our online calculator at extramilest.com/hr-calculator
"My resting heart rate varies day to day"	Use a 7-day average of morning measurements for more stability
"My zones still don't match how I feel"	Your true max HR may differ from estimates; consider a field test

Advantages

- More accurate than simple percentage of max HR by factoring in resting heart rate
- Reflects current fitness level (as fitness improves, resting HR decreases)
- Accounts for individual cardiovascular differences
- Adjusts naturally as fitness improves

Limitations

- Still requires knowing maximum heart rate
- Requires accurate resting heart rate measurement
- Resting heart rate fluctuates based on stress, hydration and sleep quality
- More complex calculations than simpler methods

Method 6: Laboratory Testing

Quick Start: Schedule testing at a sports performance laboratory for the most precise, personalized heart rate zones based on your unique physiology.
   Laboratory testing provides:

- **Lactate threshold testing:** measures your blood lactate levels as intensity increases
- **VO_2 max testing:** analyzes oxygen consumption and carbon dioxide production
- **Detailed, personalized heart rate zones:** based on your unique physiology

Who It's Best For

- Competitive runners seeking maximum performance
- Athletes who haven't found success with other methods
- Those with unusual physiological responses to exercise
- Runners wanting the most accurate data possible

A Real-World Example: Jennifer's Precision Advantage

Jennifer, a 62-year-old competitive age-group runner, was frustrated with lack of progress. The MAF Formula placed her aerobic pace at 118, which felt absurdly easy.

Laboratory testing revealed her actual aerobic threshold was at 132 bpm, far higher than the MAF Formula predicted. By adjusting her zones upward based on actual physiology, she trained more effectively. Six months later, she set a 9-minute improvement on her marathon PR and qualified for the Boston Marathon.

Troubleshooting Tips: Laboratory Testing

Challenge	Solution
"My test results seem off"	Ensure you're well rested, hydrated and not ill on test day; consider retesting if results don't make sense
"Laboratory testing is expensive"	Consider it a one-time investment; retest only every 6–12 months or after significant fitness changes
"I can't find a testing facility near me"	Some sports medicine clinics and universities offer testing; alternatively, combine other methods for best approximation
"My zones changed dramatically from my previous approach"	Transition gradually to new zones; trust the process and evaluate how you feel

Advantages

- Most accurate and tailored to your physiology
- Precisely identifies aerobic and anaerobic thresholds
- Provides insights into metabolic health
- Eliminates guesswork in training

Limitations

- Costly ($100–$200+ per session)
- Testing involves maximal effort with some injury risk
- Results affected by temporary conditions (fatigue, stress, hydration)
- Requires regular retesting as fitness evolves

Combining Methods for Better Results

Many successful runners combine methods, for example:

- Use the MAF Method for base-building periods, then heart rate reserve for race-specific training
- Use laboratory testing annually for precise zones, then compare with the talk test
- Use a heart rate monitor for training but rely on nose breathing when you want to run by feel or your device isn't available

Example: James, an ultrarunner in our training program, used MAF training (138 bpm) for three months, then had lab testing to confirm his aerobic threshold at 140 bpm. Now he uses his monitor for precise training but regularly performs "talk test checks" to ensure perceived effort matches heart rate.

Next Steps

1. **Choose a method** that matches your experience level, equipment and goals
2. **Track your results** by recording heart rate and pace during runs
3. **Adjust as needed** because no formula is perfect for everyone
4. **Be patient** and remember that improvements may take 4 to 8 weeks to become noticeable

> **TRY THIS:** Set your watch to beep when your heart rate goes above your target zone. See how often it goes off.

Next Steps: Beyond the Numbers

Heart rate training is ultimately about developing body awareness, not just following numbers. As you practice these methods, you'll develop an intuitive sense of effort that will serve you in training and racing.

Ask yourself:

1. Which of these methods feels most sustainable for my lifestyle?
2. Am I willing to trust the process even if it means slowing down initially?
3. How might training at the right intensity change my enjoyment of running?

Chapter Summary

- Multiple valid methods exist for determining your training zones, from equipment-free to laboratory testing.
- Combining methods often provides the most complete picture.
- Consistency with your chosen method matters more than which method you choose.

In the next chapter, we'll explore how to implement heart rate training in your daily runs, including my personal journey and practical tips for making this approach work for you.

5
Implementing Heart Rate Training Successfully

The best advice I can give is to be patient. Give yourself a timeline that's realistic ... Our bodies change gradually over time, but when we create those slow changes, those are the significant changes.

—Mark Allen (6x World Champion Ironman)

Now that you understand different methods for calculating your heart rate zones, let's talk about how to implement this knowledge practically. In this chapter, I'll share my own journey with heart rate training and offer guidance on how to make it work for you.

My Personal Journey with Heart Rate Training

When I first started using heart rate training, I was shocked at how slow I needed to run to stay in my target zone on aerobic runs. On hills, I often had to walk to keep my heart rate down. It felt embarrassing as other runners passed me. But I trusted the process.

After about four weeks of consistent low heart rate training, I noticed something remarkable. I was running faster at the same heart rate. The runs that had once felt frustratingly slow were now starting to flow and feel more enjoyable. I was covering more distance with the same effort, and most importantly, I was injury-free for the first time in years.

This experience taught me a crucial lesson: our bodies adapt when given the right stimulus and adequate recovery time. By training primarily in the aerobic zone, I built a stronger cardiovascular system and more efficient muscles, which eventually translated to better performance across all running intensities.

> **REMEMBER:** If you're walking on hills during heart rate training, you're doing it RIGHT, not wrong.

The Right Heart Rate Zones for You

I recommend trying several methods to determine your optimal training intensity and comparing them to see which feels most accurate for your body. Each approach has its strengths and limitations.

Start with simple methods like the talk test (running at a pace where conversation is comfortable) or nasal breathing (breathing only through your nose). If you have a heart rate monitor, check your heart rate a few times during a conversational run to see what numbers correspond to this effort.

Personally, I've used the MAF 180 Formula successfully for years, for my runs at low intensity, and it matched closely with my laboratory test results, talk test and conversation pace. Many athletes I've worked with have had great success with the MAF Method, though others have found significant differences between lab test data and the formula.

There is no perfect way to measure your ideal training zones. Even laboratory testing has its limitations. I've personally experienced inaccurate lab results because I'd had a poor night's sleep and was under significant stress at the time, requiring me to schedule a retest. Remember that your body's responses can vary, day to day, based on many factors.

One reason I particularly value the MAF Method is that it considers your current health and fitness, adjusting your target heart rate accordingly. If you have been sick, have overtrained or are coming back from an injury, the method naturally guides you toward lower training intensities. Conversely, if you're healthy, fit and progressing consistently, your target heart rate is appropriately higher. This adaptability makes it a practical, health-first approach to training.

Getting Started with Heart Rate Training

If you're eager to implement heart rate training right away, here are three practical tips to help you begin:

1. **Start with the simplest method first:** Try the talk test on your next run, and aim to run at a conversational pace. Notice how this effort feels and, if you have a heart rate monitor, check what numbers correspond to this comfortable intensity.
2. **Be patient with the adjustment period:** Your first few weeks or months of low heart rate training may require significantly slowing down or taking walk breaks. This is normal and temporary. Trust that consistent training in the right zones will yield improvements in the coming weeks and months.
3. **Focus on consistency over intensity:** Rather than worrying about perfect numbers, aim for regular training (3–4 times weekly) primarily in your easy zones. The habit of training consistently at the right intensity will build a foundation that allows for more challenging workouts later.

Case Study
Finding Joy in the Journey:
Heidi's Running Transformation

Heidi Moreno used to have no real structure in her training. Despite being an organized person, she struggled to prioritize her mental health, focusing only on what fed her ego: work, and getting faster at running.

"When I joined the PB Program it was so refreshing to see that the first module stressed the importance of mental health," Heidi recalls. "I began journaling more and making time for meditation. I had to finally confront my poor sleeping habits. I used to feel almost pride in sleeping less because it meant I was working so hard. Now I see how toxic that mindset can be."

The transformation in her running perspective was dramatic. Instead of obsessing over numbers, Heidi learned to appreciate incremental progress. This shift was put to the test during a half-marathon.

"There was a moment in the race when I looked at my watch and realized that I wasn't going to PR or beat my time from last year even. I was already in the pain cave, fighting nausea, thirst I couldn't seem to quench and thoughts about just stopping to walk instead.

"But something unexpected happened: My legs felt fresh again! They were not fighting against me, like the rest of my body was. They were urging me to keep running and get to that finish line. So I ran, and I remembered to smile like Kipchoge does, with full awareness that I was not going to PR."

The training she had done was paying off. "All those runs from the summer were showing up during those last 3 miles, where I passed so many runners as I said my mantras aloud and told myself, 'I can and I will.'"

Building on this foundation, Heidi set her sights on the Los Angeles Marathon. Despite pre-race nerves that gave her "stomach panic attacks," she approached training methodically.

"I ran 15 miles (24 km), my longest run yet!! I couldn't believe how strong I felt! I actually had gas in the tank after 12 miles (19 km), so I sped up the last 3 miles (5 km) and cried happy tears. I'm totally seeing the benefits of low heart rate training, and I'm so incredibly grateful! No injuries and no pain, and I was able to get back to training with no issues!"

Her marathon performance exceeded her expectations: "I CRUSHED my first ever marathon! It took me 6:08:20, but honestly, I enjoyed EVERY single mile. I was in a meditative state in pure bliss and happiness! I never once hit the wall! I even finished in negative splits!"

Most impressively, Heidi didn't stop there. Just months after her marathon debut, she completed her first ultramarathon, a 50K run in the Mojave Desert.

"I loved it so much I even designed a tattoo and got it done to remember this huge achievement! The other great thing was that I can tell I'm really locking into my fueling skills. I never bonked (became functionally depleted of glycogen) or had any cramps. I was just a slow tortoise in the Mojave Desert."

> Heidi's journey exemplifies how her transformation is not just physical, but mental. She sums it up perfectly: "I have learned how to change my perspective to become a healthy and happy runner."

Full Episode:
extramilest.com/93

Finding Joy in the Process

Remember that the goal isn't just to improve your running performance but to find sustainable joy in the process. By training at the right intensities, you'll discover that running can become meditative rather than a constant struggle. You'll finish runs feeling energized rather than depleted, and you'll build fitness that lasts rather than experiencing the roller coaster of progress and injury.

In the next chapter, we'll explore how to incorporate these heart rate zones into a balanced training plan that optimizes both intensity and recovery. But for now, I encourage you to experiment with the methods we've discussed, find what works best for your body and embrace the patience required for long-term success.

Chapter Summary

- Heart rate training requires patience and consistency, especially initially when you might need to significantly slow your pace or incorporate walking.
- Use methods like the talk test, nose breathing or MAF Formula to find your optimal training zones, but always prioritize how your body feels over strict numbers.
- Expect an adaptation period with gradual improvements over weeks and months, rather than immediate results.

6
Balancing Volume and Intensity in Training

Every run used to feel like a battle for me. I thought pushing harder would make me faster. My first marathon in 2007 was a massive struggle. I swore I would never run a second one. The training approach I'd taken left me completely exhausted, injured and frustrated.

It took years for me to realize that improvement wasn't about training harder but maintaining a proper balance between intensity, volume and recovery. I needed to train smarter, not just harder.

Now that we've discussed training zones and how to implement them, let's address how to balance training intensity, volume and recovery to become a stronger and healthier runner.

The Three Dials of Training

Think of your training as having three adjustable dials that you can turn up or down.

THE THREE DIALS OF TRAINING

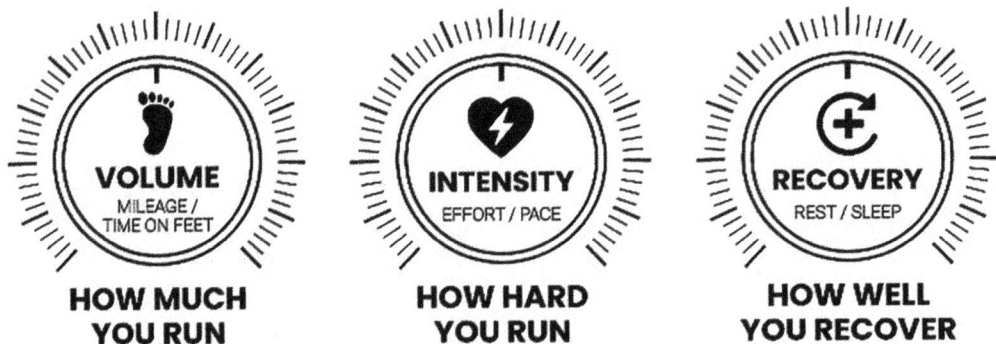

TRAINING IS A BALANCE TO AVOID INJURIES AND BURNOUT

The magic happens when these three dials are balanced properly for YOUR unique situation. Finding the right balance is essential for progress, injury prevention and enjoyment.

The Intensity Dial: Finding Your Sweet Spot

Think of your training intensity like a volume knob with three key settings.

> **Easy (Zones 1–2): Your Foundation**
> **For recreational runners, I suggest at least 80% of your training happens here.**

- **Feel:** Between 3 and 5 out of 10 effort level
- **Talking:** Relaxed enough to chat comfortably with a running partner
- **Recovery days (Zone 1):** Extremely easy (2 or 3 out of 10)
- **Regular easy runs (Zone 2):** Purposeful but sustainable for hours (4 or 5 out of 10)

Many runners make the big mistake of running too fast on easy days. If you're breathing hard or can't talk in complete sentences, you're going too fast. You should finish feeling like you could do it all comfortably again. If it feels like you're running too slowly, you're probably at just the right pace.

Moderate (Zone 3): The No Man's Land
This "tempo" effort feels comfortably hard:

- **Feel:** 6 or 7 out of 10 effort level
- **Talking:** Short phrases between breaths
- **Purpose:** Builds endurance and lactate clearance
- **Warning:** Many runners spend too much time here

Zone 3 runs help build endurance but should be used strategically and not as your default everyday pace. This is the no man's land where many recreational runners spend too much time. It's too hard for optimal aerobic development but not hard enough for maximum performance gains.

Hard (Zones 4–5): The Sharp Edge
These zones represent high-intensity work:

- **Feel:** 7 to 9 out of 10 effort level
- **Talking:** Limited to just a few words at a time
- **Zone 4 (Threshold):** Hard but controlled (8 out of 10 effort)
- **Zone 5 (Maximum):** Near-maximum effort (9 to 10 out of 10 effort)
- **Examples:** Interval workouts, hill repeats, race-pace efforts

These intensities deliver powerful training stimuli but require significant recovery. They're like spice in your training. A little goes a long way, and it's easy to overdo it. On the other hand, it's also easy to avoid, given the challenge. This is why many runners prefer spending time in the moderate zone.

Finding Your Ideal Training Approach

When determining your ideal training approach, consider two effective approaches based on your goals, health and lifestyle:

- **Aerobic Base Period (100% Low Intensity):** Spend at least 8 to 12 weeks doing only low-intensity runs before introducing higher-intensity work. This builds your aerobic foundation and significantly reduces injury risk.
- **The 80/20 Approach:** Alternatively, structure your training with about 80%–90% low-intensity and 10%–20% medium- to high-intensity work.

The MAF Method: Build Your Aerobic Base

I often recommend a pure aerobic base phase for runners new to the sport, those returning from injury or burnout or those who've hit a plateau in their performance. This involves at least 8 to 12+ weeks using the MAF Method (see Chapter 5).

During this phase, you shift to a 100/0 distribution, where all your runs stay at sustainable intensities. This is about accumulating volume your body can absorb and adapt to. I like the health and fitness modifications of the MAF Method.

This approach has several benefits:

- It builds your aerobic foundation from the ground up
- It's gentle on your body and mind, reducing injury risk while your body adapts
- It teaches you patience and proper pacing

During base building, if you feel like running at higher intensity from time to time, or running with a friend or a group without slowing down, go for it. I understand the joy and social component in training is super important. However, I suggest not overdoing this and listening to how your body responds. Injury-prone and overtrained athletes should be extremely careful with high heart rate workouts.

Profile Example

John, a 52-year-old runner and member of our Personal Best Program, had recurring calf injuries and couldn't break the sub-2-hour half-marathon barrier. We committed to three months of strict MAF training at below 138 bpm. By week 10, his easy pace had improved by 1:20 per mile (50 sec per km) at the same heart rate. He also finished a 10-mile (16-km) training run without injuries for the first time in years. Several months later, he ran an injury-free 1:52 half-marathon.

Adding Some Intensity After Base Building

You've worked on your base. Now look for these signs that show you're ready to add some speed:

- Your pace at the same easy heart rate has noticeably improved
- You've trained consistently without injuries for at least 8 to 12 weeks
- You feel mentally eager to challenge yourself more

When you're ready, here are some beginner-friendly workouts to get you started:

- **Strides:** Short bursts of speed lasting 15-20 seconds at around 85%-90% of your maximum effort, followed by 60-90 seconds of easy jogging or walking. Aim for 4-8 repetitions after an easy run.
- **Fartlek ("Speed Play"):** During an otherwise easy run, pick a landmark (like a tree or traffic light) and run at a moderately hard effort until you reach it, then ease back to recovery pace. Try 6-10 faster segments of 30 seconds to 2 minutes throughout a 30-45-minute run.
- **Intervals:** Try shorter efforts like 200 meters at a moderately hard effort (around 7 out of 10), followed by an easy jog or walk for recovery. Start with 4-6 reps, gradually building to 8-12.
- **Progression Runs:** During the last 5-15 minutes of a regular easy run, gently increase your pace to finish slightly faster. This teaches your body to maintain good form while fatigued.

To reduce injury risk, ensure you have easy days surrounding your high-intensity days.

The 80/20 Approach: Finding the Right Balance

Dr. Stephen Seiler's research shows that most successful elite endurance athletes across different disciplines do about 80% of their training at low intensity and 20% at moderate to high intensity, and in some cases, 90% low intensity and 10% moderate to high intensity. This balance helps build a strong aerobic foundation while providing targeted stimulus to improve performance.

The Volume Dial: How Much Should You Run?

The "right" training volume depends on your goals, experience and recovery capacity. Even more importantly, it depends on the time you realistically have available, and your body's tolerance for running stress.

Here's an example of training volume breakdown by athlete type:

For Health and Longevity:

- Train **3-4 hours per week** in Zone 2 (aerobic intensity)
- Include a small portion (**10%-20%**) of higher intensity work
- Benefits: improved cardiovascular health, insulin sensitivity, fat oxidation and brain function

For Recreational Athletes Seeking Performance Gains:

- Aim for **4-6 hours per week** (approximately **25-30 miles, or 40-50 kilometers**)
- Follow the 80/20 principle to balance improvement and injury prevention

For Competitive Recreational Athletes:

- Consider **6-10 hours per week** (approximately **30-50 miles, or 50-80 kilometers**)
- Maintain **80%** in Zones 1 and 2, with targeted higher-intensity sessions
- Ideal for Boston Marathon qualification or significant personal records

In my coaching, I've noticed some runners actually undertrain rather than overtrain. If you're struggling to increase running volume, consider adding 2-4 hours of low-intensity cross-training weekly (walking, cycling, swimming, elliptical). This builds aerobic capacity without additional joint stress.

Example Training Schedule

For a recreational runner training about 5 hours per week, this might mean 4 hours of easy, conversational running and 1 hour of moderate- to high-intensity work.

Here's what that might look like:

Example of a Weekly Training Schedule for a Recreational Runner

Day	Training	Intensity Zone	Duration
Monday	Rest or very easy cross-training	Recovery	–
Tuesday	Easy run	Zone 2	30–45 min
Wednesday	High-intensity session*	Zone 4 with Zone 1 recoveries	45–60 min
Thursday	Recovery run	Zone 1	45 min
Friday	Rest or very easy cross-training	Recovery	–
Saturday	Long run	Zone 2 (last 15–20 min in Zone 3)	60–90 min
Sunday	Easy run	Zone 2	45–60 min

*Example high-intensity session: Warm-up, then 6 x 3 minutes in Zone 4 with 2-minute Zone 1 recoveries, followed by cooldown.

Why does this 80/20 balance work so well? When you keep most runs easy, you build aerobic capacity while limiting fatigue and injury risk. The strategic hard sessions provide stimulus for additional performance gains.

Free Training Schedules

- Download free training schedules at florisgierman.com/training-schedules

The Recovery Dial: Where the Magic Happens

Many runners miss the fact that fitness gains happen during recovery. Workouts create stress, but in recovery your body adapts and gets stronger. If you shortchange recovery, you limit your improvement and increase injury risk.

THE ADAPTATION CURVE

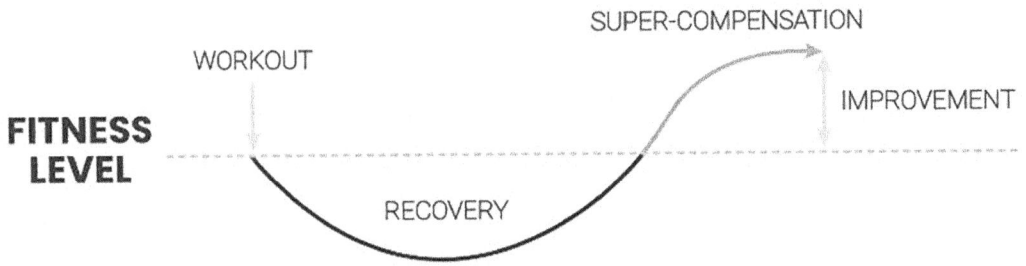

Pay attention to your body

Your body and mind constantly provide feedback to guide your training. Learning to interpret this feedback is perhaps the most valuable skill you can develop as a runner.

Green Lights (signs you can handle your current training load):

- Waking up feeling refreshed and eager to run
- Stable or decreasing resting heart rate
- Steady improvement in easy pace at the same heart rate
- Good energy throughout the day

Yellow/Red Lights (signs you need more recovery):

- Persistent fatigue or heavy legs that don't improve after an easy day
- Trouble sleeping despite being tired
- Elevated resting heart rate (especially if 5+ beats above normal)
- Decrease in sex drive
- Irritability, low motivation or declining performance

Ignoring the warning signs

I pushed myself with 80-mile (129-km) training weeks for my first 100-mile (161-km) run and ignored several warning signs: disrupted sleep, elevated resting heart rate and unusual irritability. Instead of backing off, I logged back-to-back long runs that left me with a respiratory infection that required more than a week of complete rest.

Key strategies for recovery include:

- **Sleep:** Aim for 7–9 hours of quality sleep. Athletes getting less than 7 hours have nearly double the injury rates.
- **Nutrition and Hydration:** Stay hydrated throughout the day and focus on whole foods rich in nutrients.
- **Active Recovery:** Gentle movement like easy jogging, cycling or swimming can boost recovery.
- **Rest Days:** Don't be afraid to take full rest days. These aren't "wasted" training days. They're essential for getting stronger. Walking is still a great way to keep moving on rest days.

The Mindset of Balance

Remember that consistency beats occasional high volume. Find the volume that fits your life and allows you to train consistently. Be flexible. Train smart. Recover deliberately. Your future running self will thank you.

Next Steps

Reflect on the following questions:

1. Which of the three dials (intensity, volume, recovery) do you tend to emphasize most in your current training?
2. Which dial do you most often neglect or minimize?
3. What one small adjustment could you make this week to create better balance?
4. How might focusing more on recovery improve your running experience?
5. What would an ideal training week look like for you, considering your life constraints?

Chapter Summary

- Training volume and intensity should match your goals, experience level and recovery capacity.
- Consistency with moderate volume produces better results than occasional high-volume training with frequent interruptions.
- Find the balance that works best for your unique situation.

PART 2
Elite Athletes in Conversation

One of the most exciting things about running and improving your health is that there's always something new to learn about your body, your mind, training, racing and daily life. Over the past decade, I've had the chance to talk to some of the best athletes in the world, getting firsthand insight into how they approach training and competition.

Most of us don't have the time or lifestyle of elite runners, but there's still a lot we can learn from them. These athletes put serious thought into every aspect of their training, recovery and racing. In this section, I've selected some of the most insightful conversations I've had with athletes like Eliud Kipchoge, Courtney Dauwalter, Kilian Jornet and Taylor Knibb.

I've always aimed to ask questions that are just as relevant today as they will be ten years from now, like how they push through tough moments, what mistakes they've learned from, and what advice they have for runners looking to improve. These are athletes I have a lot of respect for, and I'm excited to share their lessons with you in their own words. In a few instances, I have lightly edited these conversations for the purpose of clarity. Otherwise, these transcriptions reflect the discussions as they happened.

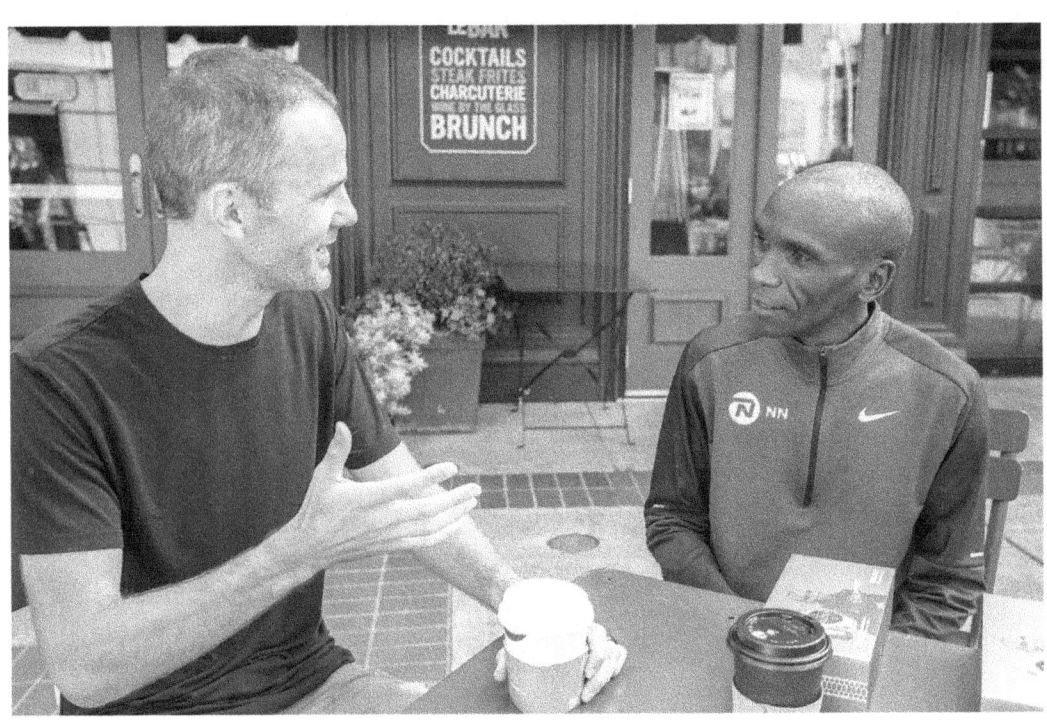

A conversation with Eliud Kipchoge about the role of consistency and joy in running and life.

Eliud Kipchoge on Consistency and Joy

"Start training and finish. Enjoy. When you're running, please enjoy. Just run and finish. And all in all, day after day, week after week, month after month, you will improve. One tip I'll tell you to improve for running is to walk your talk. It's to be consistent in training and dedicate yourself fully. Improvement goes hand in hand with dedication."

Eliud Kipchoge stands as the greatest marathoner in history—the only human to break the 2-hour barrier and a two-time Olympic gold medalist in the marathon. Born and raised in rural Kenya, he first dominated track racing, winning Olympic medals and World Championship gold in the 5000m, before transitioning to the marathon. He's since won 15 of 18 marathons, including a world record 2:01:09 that stood until 2023. Despite accomplishing everything in the sport, Kipchoge remains humble and down-to-earth, a visionary and symbol of endurance, discipline and excellence who sets a towering standard. His philosophical approach embodies the belief that "no human is limited," inspiring countless runners in both training and life.

Connect:
instagram.com/kipchogeeliud

Full Episodes:
extramilest.com/47
extramilest.com/83

Consistency Fuels Progress

Do you have any advice for recreational athletes looking to improve in their running?

The best tip is consistency. The more you are consistent, the faster improvement comes. Try to create time to just go out. The more you take control of what you are doing, the better. Be disciplined to follow the plan. It's about a decision. You create time. You just wake up in the morning and go. If you don't feel like going, just try to control your mind. That's the only way to be consistent.

You come across as a very Zen-like, calm person. How are you able to be so calm and controlled, even in quite stressful situations sometimes?

I believe that this world is full of criticisms and compliments, and that's what makes me calm. I believe that the more you are calm, the more you can make nice decisions. I believe that when you are calm, you can think in a good way, you can control what's in your hand and you can plan for the next move.

Be Methodical in Your Training

What are your thoughts on journaling?

They say, "Write it down, and you'll remember." I do a lot of journaling. I really journal my training and what I'm reading. I write the training program of the day, what I'm doing for that day. I write down my exercises, morning run, evening run, biking, massage. That's what I'm recording. I don't want to miss anything. I also record what shoes I'm using.

Looking at your training, what's the most important part of training for you? Is it the long run, volume, intensity?

Every part of training is important. Long runs help me condition my body to sustain high speeds for a long time. Intensity and intervals train my muscles to run fast. Recovery runs allow my muscles to recover. Every type of run is crucial.

Love What You Do and Don't Fear Failure

You have a lot of fun when you're running, right? I often see you smiling when you're running, and that is such an important part of training and racing as well.

Yes, that's love. That's loving what you do. They say in science there is no perfection, but if you love what you do, that's next to perfection.

What advice do you have for other runners out there when their training runs or their races are not going according to plan?

I'll give you an example of horse racing. You can go to training with the horse every day, and the horse is running very fast, but during the race, you never know what will happen. A random problem can come in, and you can't perform. It's not the end of the world when you don't perform. It actually teaches you that life is about compliments and criticism. You can criticize yourself, and that's life. You can compliment yourself, and that's life.

What do you do when you experience challenges on a long run or in the middle of a race? Is there anything that you do to get through a tough spot?

I treat it as a challenge, and you know when it's a challenge, it has happened. You have no control over it, so you need to retreat, think outside the box, provide a solution and move on. What has happened is like yesterday. You can't control yesterday, but you can control what you are doing today, and you can plan for tomorrow.

Plan for Success

When you're guiding younger athletes and giving them advice, what are some of the guiding principles? Is there anything high-level that you tell them to help them improve, especially when there's big pressure or big expectations?

The first thing is that I don't sugarcoat things for young people. I tell them to set a goal and be real professionals. Know that everything is not actually an overnight event. It's step by step. I give them an example of going to the gym. If you go to the gym for ten hours, and someone else goes to the gym for six months, who will be fitter? The one who went for six months will be more fit, have lean muscles, good muscles and be more capable of meeting specific performance expectations. If you go for ten hours, you cannot do anything. So, it's step by step. It cannot happen in one night. That's why you want young people to grow in a good way, step by step.

Running for Health and Happiness

Do you have any closing thoughts for people to become stronger, healthier and happier athletes?

Improvement goes hand in hand with dedication. I would advise recreational runners to make a weekly plan, record their progress and understand their body. Get good shoes, a good heart rate monitor, and enjoy running. Day after day, week after week, month after month, you will improve.

Sport is life. It fits everyone, whether you're a graduate of kindergarten or a professional in engineering. Running is where you are free. You are not running in prison. Love running, and you'll gain a lot of energy. Running benefits the body and mind.

They say health is wealth. The only way to be wealthy is to make sure you're fit. I want to encourage everyone to really be consistent. The more they learn, the more they improve their lives. Whether it's children going to school or people working, the more you're fit, the more you can sit for long; the more you're fit, the more you can perform at work.

If you compare someone who isn't fit with someone who is, those are two people who can produce different results. So, let's encourage health. Let's run and enjoy this world. Don't wait to enjoy your life. Run, feel that sweetness, take a shower and then go to work.

Favorite Takeaways from Our YouTube Community

@jonathansandberg5983 – "Enjoy, when you are running, please enjoy." It seems like Kipchoge is always relaxed and smiling when he runs. It's funny to me that a lot of people view running as a kind of masochistic torture, but for me, it's the best part of my day. It's so important to take pleasure in it.

@Run8va – I love the health-is-wealth sentiment. I started my running journey overweight and struggling to run for more than 30 seconds to a minute to finishing over 100 marathons and losing 70+ pounds in the process. Invest in yourself!

@twinpinescoloradocabin4879 – Great interview! My biggest takeaway was the following quote, "In running and in life, it's important to grow slowly, to be patient, but above all, be consistent in training."

@belliiahmed – Eliud inspired me to run, and as he said, I always try to listen to my body and take notes for my training to improve it. And of course my favorite quote of his is "No Human Is Limited."

Courtney Dauwalter on Mastering the Pain Cave

"Every morning, I check in with my legs, body, emotions and stress levels while drinking coffee. There's no real system to it: no data, no heart rate monitoring; it's just about noticing how I feel. If something feels off, I adjust my training accordingly. It lets me listen to my body and adjust when necessary, rather than forcing things. There are so many ways to approach it, and we all have to figure out what works for us."

Courtney Dauwalter, widely regarded as the greatest ultrarunner of all time (GOAT), has redefined the limits of human endurance with her incredible achievements, all while staying humble and never taking herself too seriously. She accomplished what many thought impossible, winning three of the most iconic ultraraces in just nine weeks. She set a course record at Western States, followed by a record-breaking performance at Hardrock 100, and capped it off with a victory at the Ultra-Trail du Mont-Blanc (UTMB) 100-mile race. Known for her humor, positive vibes and down-to-earth nature, Courtney is not only an extraordinary athlete but also a role model who inspires the running community to push their limits with a smile.

Connect:
courtneydauwalter.com

Full Episode:
extramilest.com/88

Achieving the Impossible

What was your first marathon experience like?

I thought 26.2 miles (42 km) was impossible. I was really scared. I stood at the start line among all these people, thinking, "This is it. I might not make it." But I finished! It was hard. My legs and feet hurt, but I couldn't believe I made it. It was a cool experience. It's that fear of the unknown that can hold us back, but once you do it, it opens up so many more possibilities.

What were some mistakes and lessons you learned in your first 31-mile (50K), 50-mile (80K) and 100-mile (161K) races?

Oh man, I made so many mistakes and still do! After the marathon, I thought, "What else can I do?" I didn't know ultraraces existed. My biggest mistakes were not training on trails and not figuring out nutrition. I lived in the city, so I ran city blocks and hoped it would translate to trail running. It doesn't. I fell a lot. My knees, hands and elbows were always covered in scabs. Nutrition was a whole other learning curve, figuring out how to eat while running. It took years of trial and error. Eating while running was foreign to me. I had to learn how to fuel while exerting myself for hours, and it's something you have to practice. Everyone is different in what works for them. You really have to experiment and figure out what your body needs.

Master the Pain Cave with Positivity

Let's talk about the pain cave. How has your approach to discomfort evolved over time?

Early on, I used to fear the pain cave. I thought of it as a place to avoid for as long as possible, but then I realized it was just a story I was telling myself. I flipped the script and now see it as the place where the real work happens. The harder the race, the more I visualize going into the pain cave and chiseling away at the struggle, knowing it's making me better. Mantras help me get through those tough moments. My go-to is "You're fine. This is fine. Everything is fine." But I've also used "believe," "be patient," and once even "robot, robot, robot" during the last 40 miles (64 km) of UTMB. It's about keeping the focus on the moment, on the breath, and staying relaxed.

For people who are new to trail running or ultrarunning, what advice do you have for them?

Just get out there and start small. Leave your watch at home, don't worry about pace, and enjoy being out in nature. Maybe even go with a friend, bring snacks and make it an adventure.

How do you approach recovery between big races, especially when you have multiple ultraraces close together?

I really tune in to how I'm feeling physically, mentally and emotionally. I listen to my body and am patient with the process. Sometimes it's full rest days; other times it's just walking or biking to get the blood flowing. The key is not rushing back into running.

Set Big Goals and Learn from Your Failures

You've chased so many big goals, and sometimes you've achieved them, sometimes you haven't. What are your thoughts on setting big goals and dealing with the potential for failure?

I think setting big goals is essential. You want to be pushing yourself and aiming for things that feel out of reach. Failure is always a possibility, but that's part of the excitement. When you fail, you learn, and when you succeed, it's even sweeter because of how hard you worked. Either way, you grow, and that's what makes it worth it. Failure is part of the process. It doesn't feel good at that moment, but it teaches you so much. It's important to let yourself feel bummed out for a little while, but then move on and take the lessons with you to the next challenge. Failure is necessary for growth. It's part of learning how to try new things and push your limits. Without failure, you wouldn't know how far you can go.

I've seen you smiling and laughing during some of your hardest races. How do you keep such a positive attitude, even in those tough moments?

I think they go hand in hand. You can be suffering and still smile. Running is something we choose to do, so even when it's hard, I try to remember how lucky I am to be out there. Sometimes it's because of the people around me, cheering or volunteering, and other times it's just knowing that these hard moments are where we grow the most.

Looking back, is there any advice you would give to your younger self, maybe to Courtney who was standing at the starting line of that first marathon?

I'd probably just tell myself to buckle up and enjoy the ride! It's going to be a lot of fun. But seriously, I'd say, just try. Go after things that seem impossible because, even if it doesn't work out the way you thought, you'll learn so much along the way. The journey is the real adventure, not the finish line.

Any closing thoughts?

Just keep showing up. Whether it's a mile, two miles or a long run, it all adds up. Be patient with the process, stay consistent and, most importantly, have fun with it. This is something we get to do, so enjoy the adventure and keep finding joy in the journey.

Favorite Takeaways from Our YouTube Community

@mlouw8218 – My favorite takeaway was flipping the script on pain and discomfort from avoidance to "This is where I get to learn and grow." I think this could be applied to so many different areas of life.

@Bibs123 – Like Courtney, I'm a former teacher. My biggest takeaway from her is that she listens to her body each day to decide how hard to train. I think we get into the mindset that we must stick to the training plan, when actually our body should be our gauge on what run occurs on a particular day.

@kathrynhilder9609 – Loved this chat. Thank you! I think the best takeaway for me was keep the joy; it's supposed to be fun! I always try to remember that I GET to run; I don't HAVE to run. Courtney is an absolute gem of a human.

@cindyscott8470 – My takeaway that I have heard many times from her is "Try, you gotta try." This is huge, someone really powerful handing over a key that deflects fear. "Just try"!

@Kelly_Ben – It was great to hear a GOAT like her say that consistency, even a mile or two, is key. As an ultrarunner who works 60+ hours a week on my feet, it's easy to convince myself to skip runs. Consistency is my nemesis. This is a fabulous reminder that even 10–20 minutes can move me towards my goals.

Kilian Jornet on Adaptability and Intensity

"If you do one very hard session, the body will be stressed and then return to normal. However, if you repeat that hard session after a few days, and again after a few more days, the body will adjust and establish a new level of stability. It's not about one session; it's about the repetition of hard sessions throughout the year that leads to adaptations."

Kilian Jornet is widely regarded as the greatest mountain and ultrarunner of all time. Born in the Pyrenees and raised in a mountain hut, he developed a deep connection to nature that has shaped his life. His accomplishments include multiple victories at UTMB, wins at Western States and Hardrock 100, climbing Mount Everest twice in a single week without supplemental oxygen, and completing the Alpine Connections project where he climbed all 82 4,000-meter peaks in the European Alps in just 19 days. Beyond his physical feats, Kilian is celebrated for his thoughtful approach to training, emphasizing understanding one's physiology, maintaining consistency and finding joy in the process.

Connect:
instagram.com/kilianjornet

Full Episodes:
extramilest.com/51
extramilest.com/52

Training Intensity and Common Mistakes

You've talked about various ways to measure training intensity. How do you approach this in your own training, especially with the challenges of mountain terrain?

When we look at training intensity, it's about understanding the metabolic work you're doing. There are many ways to measure that: heart rate, lactate, the oxygen-CO_2 ratio and so on. Some are much harder to measure daily, like oxygen and CO_2 ratios. Lactate is easier on a track but almost impossible in the mountains. Heart rate is possible to measure all the time, so I mostly use that on a daily basis. However, when determining my zones, I don't rely solely on heart rate. I link what I'm looking for in the session with the type of metabolic activation I want or the adaptation I'm seeking. Some zones relate more to heart rate, others to breathing, and some to how I feel.

For example, in my Zone 1, I'm not looking at heart rate because it can be very altered, especially in the lower ranges. I'm mostly looking for a pace where I feel like I'm recovering, where I'm not working hard, and I can breathe naturally without needing to breathe through my mouth. That's my Zone 1. It's about understanding the goal of the session in terms of adaptations and then matching that with the appropriate zone. Over the years, you learn to read this by feel, but sometimes it's more related to lactate or heart rate, and while you can measure it on specific days with tests, it's impossible to do so daily.

What are some common training intensity mistakes you see runners make?

I think the most common mistake is that people go too fast. What we call regenerative or easy running, which would be the classic Zone 1, is almost never done properly. People are often running in Zone 2 or even Zone 3 during what's supposed to be an easy run. This means they're not able to recover from the hard sessions, and when they attempt a hard session, they can't go hard enough. As a result, all their training ends up in the same area because they're too tired to push themselves properly. In general, easy means easy. It doesn't matter if you're running at 6 or 7 kilometers an hour (14–16 minutes per mile). It's not about speed. It's about making your body move, allowing some adaptations and recovering well so you can push hard during the challenging sessions.

Another common mistake is not considering all the different stresses on the body. We often think of a workout as just the training session, which places a stress of, say, 2 on the body. Then we plan the next hard session based on that number 2, but we don't account for other stresses, work, family or other factors that might add up to an 8. We really need to take all these things into account when planning the week or short cycles of training.

Adaptability and Consistency

I've noticed that some athletes are glued to a training schedule instead of adapting it based on the challenges that come up. How important is flexibility in your approach?

People often stick to the plan because the plan is like the dream. They think, "This is what will make me good," but reality is very different. We need to be able to adapt the plan. There are tools to help, like tracking how you feel or heart rate variability, but it's tough to measure how much these other stresses have affected you. If you consider heart rate variability, mood, how you're feeling, muscle tiredness, body fatigue and sleep quality together, you can understand how ready you are for a session. That's very important for daily training.

Many times, we think, "I cannot miss that session," but remember that adaptations never come from just one session. The body will always try to return to balance, to homeostasis.

What training aspects do you think are most underrated that everyone should pay more attention to?

In general, we tend to focus a lot on those big sessions or "hero weekends" where we want to train a lot and push ourselves hard. However, training isn't just about making big efforts and then being destroyed for a week. It's about consistency. Find what you can do sustainably; something you can manage week after week. That will lead to much more improvement than having a huge week or weekend of training if you can't sustain it.

When it comes to training itself, we often focus on the metabolic work of hours, distance and similar metrics, but there are other aspects we need to consider. These include how we breathe, the technical aspects of the race, our strategy and the muscular aspects of running, whether uphill, downhill or on the flat. It's not just about thinking, "I need to do two hours at this speed," but also about how we are running, pacing ourselves, eating and hydrating during training. All these aspects around the metabolic side are very important.

Tracking Progress and Journaling

You carefully track your training in a journal, similar to what Eliud Kipchoge does. Can you tell me more about your approach to journaling and why you find it valuable?

I think it's important to understand what's happening and where adaptations occur. Trusting our memory is unreliable because it often only remembers the good moments. We tend to think "Last season, I was feeling better, and my sessions were way better," but that's not always true. Journaling allows you to look back realistically and see exactly what was happening.

My journaling has evolved a lot over the years. I started recording every day since 2006. Initially, I didn't measure distance because I was training in the mountains, and distance wasn't an important metric for me. Now it is. I measured volume, elevation and time, but I also noted the terrain because it makes a big difference. I recorded intensity and subjective things like how I was feeling. I also loved to note where I was training, what place I was in, and any travel, sickness or other factors. When you look back, you can understand patterns: why you were strong at a certain time, why an injury occurred or how a small pain developed or disappeared. Journaling means you can look back realistically, seeing exactly why and how things happened. It's crucial because our memory isn't always reliable.

Do you have any advice for recreational runners looking to start journaling?

The biggest challenge is consistency. You might start by taking detailed notes but then give up after a week or a month. It's like training. You need to find the load that fits you. You can't expect to do more than what's realistic. If you can only record how you felt each day, it's much better to do that consistently than to measure everything one day and then stop.

With today's tools, it's super easy. The watch records everything for you: distance, elevation, intensity. You can use apps that sync with your watch, so you don't have to worry about those details. I suggest focusing on feelings or sensations. It's not only useful but also beautiful to read later. Writing about where you were, who you were with and the weather, for example, adds emotional feedback that's as important as the data.

Finding Balance and Motivation

How has failure helped you grow as an athlete, especially with the ambitious goals you set?

Failure is crucial. It's where you learn the most. Success often doesn't teach you much, but failure makes you analyze what went wrong and how to improve. Early in my career, failure often led to frustration, especially with technical issues in skiing. But over time, I realized that a race or project is just part of the journey, not the whole story. It's important to focus on what you learn from the process, not just the outcome. The result is just one form of validation, but not the only one. By focusing on the process, you can better understand and benefit from failure, rather than being upset or obsessed with the result.

What advice would you give to recreational runners looking to become stronger, healthier and happier athletes?

I think it's all about motivation and being happy with what you do. We train because we love it, not because it's an obligation. Especially for young athletes, the focus should be on the process, not just the goals. You need to love training, being outside and doing the workouts.

Find what truly motivates you. For some, it's the community and training with friends. For others, it's being in the mountains and enjoying the landscape. Make sure your training environment aligns with what you love. Focus on enjoying the process, and the results will follow. If you focus solely on the results, you might not achieve what you want.

What matters is being consistent, whether it's running one day every week, two days or three days. Just be consistent. This consistency will make you better because you'll sustain the training and create routines that connect you more to the sport.

How do you approach strength training, mobility and cross-training? Any advice for those with limited time?

I do a lot of cross-training, especially skiing, for six months of the year. When recovering, I prefer activities like scrambling or climbing, which are technical and slow, helping with both mobility and strength. I don't usually train in a gym, but I focus on outdoor activities that naturally work different muscle groups. If I have a specific issue, like a shoulder injury, I'll do targeted strength exercises.

For recreational runners, I suggest finding fun activities like climbing, mountain biking or snow sports, which build strength and mobility. This approach makes training enjoyable and can easily involve the whole family, making it more sustainable and less of a chore.

Any closing thoughts that you want to share?

I think we sometimes put a lot of weight on what we are doing, like training and competitions. We need to remember at the end of the day that we are doing this because we love it, and that's the most important thing. Don't forget when you are suffering, when you are obsessed about the thing, just like, "Okay, why am I doing this in the first place?" It's because I love it, and I have the health to do it, and I have the possibility of doing it. If it goes wrong, I'm still doing something that is amazing, that I love.

Favorite Takeaways from Our YouTube Community

@titosinha – When Kilian said the body always gravitates toward balance and that adaptations don't happen after one session but many, many sessions, this resonated with me. So when the body is telling me to take it easier or slower, it's okay, and to listen to it rather than being rigid in following a plan.

@chadhawkinsart – I love his last comment. "Enjoy the process more than the goal." I'm training to qualify for the Boston Marathon and I'm a very goal-oriented person. It's a great reminder to soak up the process and not just the goal.

@kirstyvanniekerk8680 – "A training session is not a race"— something we so easily forget. Potent reminder <3

@RunwithSung – This was a fantastic interview. "Plan is the dream. But plan to reality is very different. We need to be able to adapt to the plan (reality?)." (I laughed at myself when he talked about plan vs. reality. I think all runners can resonate with this. Ha!)

@LucaBaldassarre – "Learn who you are" to understand how to train, race, eat and recover. Kilian did a lot of self-experimentation, and it's good that he reminds us to experiment ourselves too to learn what works and what doesn't work for each of us as different individuals.

Mark Allen on Mindset and Meditation

"Develop the ability to quiet your mind. At any point in the day, in anything you're doing, you can try to find that quiet place. As an athlete, during any training session, when the workout starts to get tough or when I'm not feeling as good as I'd hoped, and that little voice in my head begins to doubt, that's when I pull everything back. I take one breath, find that quiet place and then keep going. It only takes an instant, but the more you practice, the more it becomes the place you go almost with every breath you take."

Mark Allen is a six-time Hawaii Ironman World Champion, named the "Greatest Triathlete of All Time" by *Triathlete* magazine and the "World's Fittest Man" by *Outside* magazine. His journey was marked by perseverance, especially after multiple near-wins at Kona before his dominant streak from 1989 to 1995. Mark's success wasn't just about physical endurance but a holistic approach that combined heart rate training with Dr. Phil Maffetone and mental resilience work with shaman Brant Secunda. Today, he continues to inspire athletes through coaching, books and seminars, emphasizing the importance of training both body and mind.

Connect:
markallensports.com

Full Episode:
extramilest.com/5

A Transformative Training Approach

At the peak of your career, you ran 5:20 per mile (3:19 min/km) at an aerobic heart rate of 155 beats per minute, which blew my mind and inspired me to try heart rate training. What was that experience like initially?

When I started, the first time Dr. Phil Maffetone took me to the track and had me put on the heart monitor, my pace was 8:45 minutes per mile (5:26 minutes per kilometer). It was a shock because most of my runs were under 5:30 min/mile pace (3:25 min/km), 5:15 min/mile (3:16 min/km), 5:10 min/mile (3:13 min/km) even for a quarter mile. That was the mentality in the early '80s. Go hard all the time. This required a significant shift in approach, and it took patience. But it became one of the primary training methods that enabled me to keep progressing and get faster every year throughout my 15-year career.

How did your training approach change when you began working with Dr. Phil Maffetone?

When I began triathlon training in 1982, I came from a swimming background where the mentality was to go hard all the time. Coaches prescribed the toughest possible workouts with no focus on easy, aerobic sessions. I applied this same approach to triathlon, pushing hard on both bike and run. While this sometimes led to decent race results, it ultimately caused burnout. I experienced minor injuries requiring time off and frequently got sick after races.

Working with Dr. Phil Maffetone in 1984 introduced me to developing the aerobic system, or fat-burning system, which places much lower stress on the body compared to anaerobic training. This shift was transformative. My workouts became more consistent, race results improved, and recovery times shortened. Initially, I questioned the effectiveness because I was accustomed to feeling depleted after workouts. With this fundamental shift in mindset, I finished workouts feeling strong. It required patience, especially in running, to slow down and build my aerobic base. As my aerobic fitness improved, I became faster at a lower heart rate, with undeniable results.

How long did it take to see progression with low heart rate training?

I got faster consistently for about three years. Then the top-end speed plateaued. After three years, I was running between 5:30 min/mile (3:25 min/km) and 5:45 min/mile (3:34 min/km) at 155 beats per minute. Eventually, I reached 5:20 min/mile (3:19 min/km) at 155 beats per minute. The most significant change was in endurance. The falloff from mile to mile became minimal. Initially, starting at 5:30 min/mile (3:25 min/km), subsequent miles would slow to 5:45, 6:00 and 6:10. Over time, I could maintain consistent pacing through multiple miles with only 10 seconds total falloff. This demonstrated different aspects of fitness: raw speed versus the ability to maintain speed over time.

Cultivating the Right Mindset

In my first marathon attempt at sub-3 hours, my heart rate monitor broke, and the race was delayed 25 minutes. Despite these obstacles, staying calm was key. How do you help athletes develop this mindset?

I always tell my athletes that there is no perfect race, but you can race perfectly. That's a significant mindset shift. Whether your heart rate monitor breaks or the race is delayed, managing these challenges calmly rather than freaking out—that is racing perfectly.

I read your book *Fit Soul, Fit Body* and was fascinated by your holistic approach. What exactly is a fit soul and how can athletes work on this?

We all know what a fit body is. When you're going faster, feeling better, getting stronger and reducing body fat, those measurable markers mean you're gaining a fit body. But a fit soul is more about what's going on in your internal landscape, with your internal character.

Are you focused on fear, doubt, anger or jealousy? Or are you focused on positive qualities, like feeling peaceful in the midst of whatever's going on? Are you able to quiet your mind when challenges get tough and that voice starts saying, "No, it's not worth it. I can't do it. I should have never started this sport"? Being able to quiet your mind in those moments enables you to move through them more quickly. That's having a fit soul.

Having a fit soul also starts with trusting life itself. Many people think, "If I can achieve that goal, then I will be happy. If I can win an Ironman, then my life will be worth living." But in 1989, when I first connected with Brant Secunda, that whole dynamic shifted for me. Through studying with him and learning about Huichol shamanism, I realized that the starting point is having true trust in life that things will work out the way they're supposed to.

Going into an Ironman, I would think, "I'm the luckiest guy on the planet because look what I get to do today." It's not going to be easy, and it won't go the way I want 100% of the time, but I have the chance to truly live and express gratitude for being alive. That's having a fit soul.

Do you meditate? If so, what form of meditation works for you?

In Huichol shamanism, they don't use the word "meditate," but one of the main goals in that tradition is to develop the ability to quiet your mind. At any point in the day, in anything you're doing, you can try to find that quiet place.

I didn't wait until race day to practice this. Many athletes don't pay enough attention to their thoughts and minds. It's one thing to be quiet when nothing is going on. That's a starting point to learn how to be quiet. You can meditate, watch a sunrise or sunset, sit in the woods or watch the ocean. Immersing yourself in nature is the easiest way to quiet yourself. Then, you can start translating that sensation into finding that quiet place when you're in motion.

The real test is to see if you can do it in tough moments when things aren't going as you hoped, when it's not ideal and when you're not sitting on your couch. That's why I loved Ironman. It was not only a test of getting your body ready but also of developing the ability to find that quiet inside and use it during the race.

Building Strength and Embracing Patience

What are your recommendations for implementing strength training?

I started implementing strength training around the age of 33, when I noticed that no matter how much I swam, biked or ran, I didn't have the same snap and strength as I did in prior years. I realized that if I wanted to keep improving my performance, I needed to add strength training to my routine.

For endurance athletes, I recommend two days a week of strength training that targets all the main muscle groups. These sessions can be done in 30–45 minutes. They don't need to be long. I suggest doing slightly fewer reps with a challenging weight, aiming for 8 to 15 reps per set. If you do more than 15 reps, you typically have to lighten the weight, which shifts the focus from strength building to endurance.

Do you have any parting advice for athletes looking to improve their performance?

The best advice I can give is to be patient. Give yourself a timeline that's realistic. Everything nowadays is happening at the speed of Twitter (X), and our genetics were set up thousands of years ago. Our bodies change slowly over time, but when we create those slow changes, those are the significant changes, whether it's fitness or how we approach the world or our mindset. Be patient, enjoy the process and hook into a community of people who are trying to focus on the same things you are. It's great to do this kind of work of training and changing yourself in the company of other people.

Favorite Takeaways from Our YouTube Community

@Kelberi – "One breath and we are back to present and calm down."

@colinlancaster2196 – Mark is a special athlete and person. He is so in tune with his body and what he was trying to achieve.

@bmanley01 – Unlike the latest fad shoe, in-vogue piece of equipment or psychotherapy that must be embraced to get faster, everything said in this video then is as powerful and useful today.

Taylor Knibb on Feel over Data

"Athletically, pick something that you enjoy. You might not love it at first. You might not love it after a few times. People will tell me like, oh, I don't run, I don't like running. I'm like, well, if I take a two-week break from running, I might not love it the first day or week or month back."

Taylor Knibb is redefining endurance sports with a relentless drive, thoughtful training and joy for the sport. She's dominated the Ironman 70.3 circuit with three consecutive World Championship titles, sits at #1 in the Professional Triathletes Organisation's world rankings, and has an Olympic silver medal to her name. Taylor caught the tri bug at 11 years old watching her mom race, and she's been refining her craft ever since. After graduating from Cornell, she's built her athletic philosophy around purposeful training and holistic improvement. She works with coach Dan Lorang and movement specialist Lawrence van Lingen.

Connect:
instagram.com/taylorknibb

Full Episode:
extramilest.com/98

How has your training changed over time, and has that impacted your racing?

I think everything I do now is very purposeful. If I need to do something, I do it. If I don't, I don't. Before, my approach was more scattered. You can throw volume at an athlete, and they'll respond, but after a while, it just builds up. Fatigue sets in, and you don't know where it's coming from.

Now, my training is very specific, and it's liberating in a lot of ways. It takes a lot less mental energy because I know why I'm doing something. It's not to test me—not to prove that I'm resilient. It's about getting a stimulus with the least stress possible.

How do you go about measuring intensity, both on low-intensity days and during harder sessions, for swimming, cycling and running?

I actually got a message from Dan earlier this week because I told him, "I'm really on edge. I'm kind of frustrated. I'm really tired. I'm very emotional."

And he said, "Use the paces and everything I give you, like the bike watts and the running paces, as guidelines. But you know how it should feel. Make sure you go by feel more than anything else."

I think that's so interesting because we live in this world where we're constantly getting feedback. If you ask someone how they slept last night, how many people will say, "Oh, my sleep score was this," instead of just saying, "How did you sleep? How did it feel?"

Knowing what you know now, what advice do you have for your younger self?

Well, knowing what I know now? I wouldn't have listened to myself. So I don't think that any advice to my younger self would have been very helpful because sometimes you have to live it to learn it. You'll keep relearning lessons that you didn't quite grasp the first time.

Some things you just won't understand until you go through them, and that's the more valuable lesson. Realize what's important and why you want to do something.

I'd tell myself to just enjoy it more. I think I do for the most part, but sometimes I put extra stress and pressure on myself. And it's like, "Okay, really, how much will that change your life?" It won't. So learning how to enjoy things a bit better would have been helpful.

Let's talk about a slogan that has come up with Lawrence van Lingen: "Mastery over medals." Has your perception of that changed over the years?

I think both matter to me at this point in my career. But I was actually instructed that you have to hold your goals delicately and loosely. Because if you grip them too tightly, they'll break. Similarly, if you want medals, if you want to do well, you have to focus on mastery.

If you're only focusing on the medal, it can take you down. Medals should be a byproduct, not the entire focus.

If the idea is "I want to see how good I can be," and races are just opportunities to express yourself and your potential, then the next day, your goal and purpose aren't gone. It becomes part of your life's work.

When you hit a tough spot in a race, what goes through your mind, and how do you work through that?

You want to be prepared for the tough parts in the race because they're going to come. But at least for me, if I think about them too much beforehand, I almost feel like I'm willing them to happen.

Counting is really calming for me. It's rhythmic. It normally happens on the run. It's grounding for me.

I never really use the term "pain cave." Especially on the bike, I actually get excited about really challenging sections. My first thought is "I can get a lot of time here." It's an opportunity.

For example, in my time trial in May, there was an Olympic spot on the line. Around the 60%–80% mark of the race was the hardest part to commit to. But that's where you have to go all in. I told myself, "Taylor, this is where you're going to win it or not." And it's fun because you know that not many people are willing to make that commitment. That's where you gain time.

Do you have any high-level thoughts, recommendations or insights for endurance athletes of all levels looking to improve?

Whatever you're trying to do athletically, pick something that you enjoy. I probably don't have the same perspective as most people because my sport is everything to me. It's my job, my passion, my hobby, my form of exercise. It's a big part of my social life. But I also recognize that not everyone's situation is like mine. People have a lot of things going on in their lives.

Favorite Takeaways from Our YouTube Community

@nathanchan2334 – It's amazing how she views the "pain cave." To her, it means opportunity, something to look forward to. It really shows how much of this is mental and how you frame the experience.

@davidosolo – Behind her humility is an incredibly intelligent and authentic young woman, an extremely gifted and tough athlete. Advice to younger self: "You won't understand, unless you go through it" is definitely my favorite quote from this interview.

@woofsci – Very insightful episode, thanks Floris! Favorite lesson from this episode is the value of low-intensity training: love how Taylor emphasizes the benefits of low-intensity training for both enjoyment and recovery, leading to long-term improvement!

@ChamindaJ – Lovely conversation. Thank you, Floris. "My situation is unique to me. I will compare to me." This really resonated with me, reminding me to focus on my personal progress instead of comparing myself to others.

Ryan Hall on Strength Training

"I often ask my athletes, 'What are you craving? What do you feel like doing?' If there's a lift they love, they should start with that, then move to the next. It's important to create a positive association with the gym. You want to be doing something you enjoy, not just torturing yourself."

Ryan Hall, a legend in American distance running, holds records like a 2:04:58 marathon and a 59:43 half-marathon. Since retiring from professional running in 2016, he's transitioned into weightlifting, significantly increasing his body weight from 127 to 187 pounds. This shift has deepened his understanding of strength training, which he now emphasizes in his coaching.

Connect:
instagram.com/ryanhall3

Full Episode:
extramilest.com/54

Ease into Strength Training

A lot of recreational runners spend most of their time running and often ignore strength training and mobility. What was your initial approach to strength training, and how has that viewpoint changed over time?

I hated the gym and rushed through my workouts. I avoided upper body exercises, focusing only on core work and legs. Now, I approach things very differently for myself and my athletes. Since retiring from running, I've learned how essential heavy lifting is. If I don't lift heavy, my results suffer, even with consistency. Many distance runners avoid heavy lifting due to our small frames. It feels uncomfortable. Ironically, heavy lifting is probably what I needed the most.

I've always believed that how you do something is more important than what you do. Two athletes can follow the same training program, but one might force it and push hard all the time, while the other is confident, relaxed and lets it come naturally. The latter often responds better to training. In big training groups, top-end athletes feel good during workouts, while others push too hard and don't get the same results. They're training at an effort level they shouldn't be at.

For athletes intimidated by the gym, how do you ease them into strength training without overwhelming them?

Easing into it is super important. Anytime I take someone who hasn't been lifting, I make sure their first week feels easy, like they could do 10 more reps if they wanted to. There's a physical aspect to easing in, but also the intimidation factor of walking into a gym, especially if you feel like you don't know what you're doing.

A good solution is to work with a lifting coach at first—someone who can watch you move and take you through everything. That way, you feel much more comfortable compared to wandering into a gym and watching YouTube videos, hoping you're doing things right. It's worth it to invest in a strength coach who knows what they're doing. Ideally, you'd be lifting with other runners, too. Lifting is relative to your genetics, your body style and your sport. For example, the guys I train here in Flagstaff can't lift the same upper body weights as me because they rarely do upper body work. But if you're in a team environment, you can compare your strength to others in a way that makes sense for you. Just keep it fun. To be consistent, you need to enjoy your training.

Time of day also matters. When I was running professionally, I would lift at 5 p.m. after my second run, usually starving and low on energy. Trying to move heavy weights in that state was tough. So, knowing when your energy is at its peak is crucial. If possible, fit your weight workout into that energy window.

Embrace Intensity Variation and the Pain Cave

What are some common mistakes you see runners make, especially recreational runners?

The common mistake I see is running your easy days too hard. My dad coached me in high school and said, "Make your easy days easy and your hard days hard." It's simple but important advice. People, including myself, like to push all the time. Now with GPS, you can see your pace every second.

How do you approach and manage the discomfort during races and tough training sessions?

You have to enjoy the pain cave. You have to want to go there. A lot of people don't like being uncomfortable, but I love it. It sounds kind of sick, but if you can develop that love for the pain cave, you'll want to go there. When I was running marathons, I couldn't wait for the pain to start because that's when it gets fun. The first half was enjoyable, but I loved the grind. It's about developing a positive association with the pain. I've been doing it since I was a kid: carrying wood in the forest; pushing myself to see how much I could handle. Embrace the pain cave and learn from it.

Passion Is the Key to Success

You look comfortable when running, even when it's tough. Talk to me about relaxation in running.

Relaxation is everything. I learned this at Stanford. You have to be as relaxed as possible. If you get tight, you lose range of motion and efficiency. You want to be in control of your body: flowing, not robotic. Running should flow out of you, not be forced. Let it come to you rather than trying to look like Kipchoge or someone else. Comparison kills people in running. I wanted to look like African runners and got down to 127 pounds (57 kg), but I was terrible at that weight. You have to focus on becoming the best version of yourself, knowing your strengths and weaknesses, and having someone who knows how to program around that.

Do you have any closing thoughts on becoming a stronger, healthier and happier athlete?

Pay attention to what you love. Be excited about what you're doing. Have goals that get you out the door. Design your racing schedule around races you're excited about. Feeding your passions will make you consistent and help you enjoy what you're doing. Passion is key to success.

Favorite Takeaways from Our YouTube Community

@MadHatter-cj8bh – I like the way Ryan says "for me." He never proclaims that one thing fits all. And that's the one thing I've learned getting older: We're all different and react differently to stimuli.

@shannonsides6017 – Gahhhhh soooo many great takeaways! His energy is contagious and left me excited and inspired. Biggest takeaway was to be willing to pivot in order to stay excited about your goals.

@alexchan5042 – Do the things you enjoy to do; you will get more out of yourself.

Sally McRae on Mental Resilience

"Remember, it's your journey, and it's not supposed to look like anybody else's except yours. Appreciate the fact that you are unique, because that's going to help you enjoy the journey better."

Sally McRae is a professional ultra/mountain runner and winner of the Badwater 135, known as the toughest footrace on the planet, and the author of *Choose Strong: The Choice That Changes Everything*. Also a trainer, coach and mother of two active kids, she says she wants to live a life that shines, in which she uses what she's passionate about to reach people.

Connect:
sallymcrae.com

Full Episode:
extramilest.com/48

Cultivating a Strong Work Ethic

You balance being a professional runner for Nike, a mother, a podcast host, a coach and a business owner. How do you manage it all?

When I was growing up here in Orange County, California, we didn't have a lot. So I started working with my dad when I was seven, and I was making my own money when I was twelve. I've always worked, and I think there's something to be said about learning a work ethic in your youth.

At one point I was working at a coffeehouse and a sandwich shop, and after I would close up the shop, I would go and train in the gym for a couple of hours. So that started at a really young age, and I think this idea of juggling so much, it was just ingrained in me.

When my mom passed away, at one point, I became the guardian to my two younger siblings. When you live and operate in one way, it's all that you know. And it isn't always good because I do tend to take on too much, or I don't take care of myself all the time.

Thankfully, I have a great husband who makes me aware of that, like, "Hey, you need to go to bed; you need to rest." But the work ethic started at a very young age. I can sit and complain, or I can go and do my best with what I have, and I can go make it happen for myself. When you find the way for yourself, instead of having someone just hand it to you, oh, your reward is so much better.

When I signed as a pro, it was after I had children. I was working out two to three times a day. During their nap time, if I had to get 9 miles (14 km) in for the day, sometimes that would take me three workouts to get that in because I had two babies. And so it was believing in the work that I was doing; being relentless in that.

I don't think I have perfect balance. I think that being aware of who you are is very powerful. Being okay with accepting your weaknesses and knowing, like, this is where I struggle; this is where I need help.

My husband and I, we've been best friends since we were 18, so he knows me very well, and he has the best responses. This happened this morning. He's like, "Okay, we need to check out your to-do list. What have you written down?" And I kid you not, it was like 25 things. And he's like, "Sally, this is a to-do list for the month. We're picking 3."

I'm always a work in progress. The seasons change. When your children were babies, your life was so different. And as soon as they start potty training and feeding themselves and going to preschool, it changes all over again. And so it's being okay with adapting and bending with the seasons of life and not holding so fast to how you think it's supposed to be or how someone else's family is the perfect balance of how it should be.

Always Remember Who You Are

Many people struggle with limiting beliefs, either because they don't set high enough goals for themselves or because they've been written off by others. External factors often play a significant role in this as well. Could you share your thoughts on the role of belief and mindset, both in running and in life?

I love that you brought that up because I think, now more than ever, the outside factor is an unfortunate reason why many people don't move forward in a goal or a dream or wanting to even try something. We are now more than ever so accessible by everyone. At any given time, I can open up my phone and there's going to be dozens and dozens of messages and comments and notifications.

It's so important that we first know who we are. And it's something that we have to remind ourselves of every single day. When you look in the mirror, you have to remember who you are and realize that there's only one of you. And everything that you feel—your dreams and your goals—nobody cares about them the way that you do. And nobody ever will.

All these people who have opinions about what you can and can't do—they don't get up and actually think about your goals and whether or not you're working toward them. They're too self-focused on themselves. And so when you remember who you are and you understand that only you can make something possible and no one else can do that for you, that's really powerful. That should give you confidence.

It's important to understand that failures, letdowns, mistakes, flaws—they do not define your value. In fact, those were never supposed to be limiting factors. All of those things are supposed to help propel us to something better.

Almost like a steppingstone.

Yes, a steppingstone. We have been conditioned to believe that if I fail, that's humiliating. Everyone's gonna know, everyone's gonna see. It's like, no, it's that you just need to get better. You need to work at it. You need to train.

So when I talk to people about mindset and as it pertains more specifically to racing, you're going to hit those patches in your training and your racing, and you're going to have critics. Know what you're going to do before all of those happen. The power of quieting your mind—whether it's out on a long run, as you get up in the morning—you have those quiet moments, go over those things. I know for me, before I even stood on the start line of the Badwater 135, I had things that I knew I would tell myself. And one of the most powerful things was that every problem that arises actually isn't a problem. It's just a situation that needs a solution. It's just something that I need to take care of.

It doesn't matter whatever it is that I'm feeling or how big the problem might seem, the most important thing for me is getting to that finish line and really going after that goal with my whole heart because that's the story that I want to tell.

Embracing Your Unique Journey

You're a big advocate of strength training for runners, and you have integrated strength training from a very early age. What benefits have you experienced personally?

A couple years before I got married, I was in a bad car accident, and I got really bad whiplash. From that point on, I've always had some type of back pain. At age 22, my back was in so much pain, even just lying down hurt. I started doing Pilates because I had learned that wherever you have pain, support everything around it. So where that pain is, make everything around it stronger. So Pilates was really good for me because I wanted to make my core really strong—my abs, my glutes, everything. It was a game changer for me. And from that point on, I just continued staying with strength training.

When I entered ultrarunning in 2009, I wasn't able to find anything about how to properly train for these races. Well, if I'm going to go run around in the mountains for 50 miles (80 km), I want to have a body that can endure. Well, now here I am. Almost a decade now that I haven't been injured. And I attribute that to strength training. I'm able to hammer down a mountain so hard at the end of a 100-mile (161-km) race, and I feel good. My IT bands never hurt; my knees don't hurt; my lower back doesn't hurt.

Any final recommendations for recreational runners who want to become stronger, healthier and happier athletes?

Remember, it's your journey, and it's not supposed to look like anybody else's except yours. Take care of yourself. I can't stress that enough. I think sometimes when I talk to new athletes and beginners, they are so stressed about reaching all these goals right away. You know, they're like, "I want to get into ultrarunning. I want to run 100 miles (161 km) in three months." I'm like, "You don't need to do any of that, but you do need to appreciate and respect the journey, because there's so much that you're going to learn." So enjoy it. Take it one day at a time. When those storms come, appreciate them, because you're going to get stronger. But don't ever stop going after that dream.

Favorite Takeaways from Our YouTube Community

@russkemp1358 – My main takeaway was Sally's comments about looking in the mirror and knowing you are the only one who can go after your goals, not waiting for approval.

@oceaniccurrents – I loved how she spoke about embracing the season you are in. As a new mom I constantly was comparing this and that and how is that family able to do all this and I'm overwhelmed with just this. It's taken me a full year to just let it go and just enjoy each day for what it is.

@daveblack6367 – "I had the day that I needed." We learn best through failure. A super-inspiring interview, Floris. Thank you.

@Awhimai45 – Sally is such an inspiration! My biggest takeaway was the power of the mind. I am an older woman who loves running from New Zealand.

@ericchevalley – "How you respond to the challenge/situation is powerful" resonates with me. Each experience can be a steppingstone, especially when it doesn't go as planned.

PART 3
Optimizing Your Mind and Energy

Running isn't just about training plans and mileage; it's about how you manage your energy, mindset and ability to stay present. If you're exhausted, stressed or unfocused, no number of miles will get you where you want to go. The best runners understand that performance isn't just about pushing harder but about optimizing everything between runs.

In this section, we'll explore the tools that make the difference between simply logging miles and truly unlocking your potential. You'll learn how to create routines that set you up for success, why journaling can transform your self-awareness and how relaxation, not tension, helps you run faster and more efficiently. We'll dive into meditation, stress management and visualization techniques that can take your running to the next level.

These practices aren't just supplementary; they're foundational to becoming a stronger, healthier and happier runner. Remember that the mind leads, and the body follows.

7
How to Optimize Your Energy

Think of your energy like compound interest in a bank account. Small, consistent deposits in the right areas can lead to exponential growth over time.

The Energy Multiplication Effect

Your total energy isn't just the sum of your inputs; it's their product. Imagine rating your sleep and nutrition each on a scale of 1 to 10. If both score just 1, your energy output is tiny: $1 \times 1 = 1$. But optimize both to a 9, and suddenly you have 81 units of energy.

Take Michael, a runner in our Personal Best Program. When he first joined, his sleep scored a 4 and his nutrition a 3. After three months of focusing on these areas, he raised both to 8s. The improvement in his energy, and his running, was exponential. He went from struggling to complete workouts to setting personal best times, all while feeling more energized throughout the day.

Sleep: Your Foundation

"Sleep is the greatest legal performance-enhancing drug that most people are probably neglecting," says sleep expert Matthew Walker.

For runners, quality sleep is nonnegotiable. When I coach athletes, I often see immediate performance improvements when they prioritize these sleep practices:

- **Create a wind-down routine:** You can't just finish your workout or your daily work and expect great sleep. Read a book, go for a gentle walk, do some breathing exercises or take a bath.
- **Time your final meal wisely:** Stop eating 2–3 hours before your bedtime. This lowers your resting heart rate and gives your body time to prepare for sleep.
- **Be mindful of stimulants:** Caffeine has a 6-hour half-life. That afternoon coffee at 2 p.m.? Half of it is still in your system at 8 p.m. I don't drink caffeine after 1 p.m.
- **Maintain consistency:** Go to bed within 30 minutes of your chosen bedtime every single day.
- **Control your light exposure:** Eliminate blue light from screens an hour before bed. Switch to red and amber lights, which are less disruptive to your sleep cycle.

> **RUNNER INSIGHT:** Doug, a marathoner in our program, used to sleep only 5–6 hours a night and he was not improving in his running, even after months of trying. I suggested he aim for at least 7 hours a night by going to bed earlier. Within three weeks, his easy pace improved by more than 1 minute per mile (0:37 per km) at the same heart rate.

Fuel Your System

What you eat isn't just food; it's energy for your body. Common energy-draining nutrition mistakes I see runners make include:

- Undereating; not taking in enough calories
- Skipping post-run refueling windows
- Relying too heavily on processed foods, energy bars and drinks
- Not eating enough protein for recovery

Hydration is equally crucial. Even mild dehydration can fog your thinking and sap your energy. While most people think electrolytes are just for intense training, they're essential for daily energy and mental clarity. Keep water nearby and sip throughout the day, but don't forget about electrolyte balance.

Know Your Numbers

At least once a year, get a comprehensive blood test. I've encountered numerous athletes whose energy levels were compromised by underlying deficiencies, such as:

- Low iron levels
- Vitamin D deficiency
- Thyroid imbalances
- Hormonal issues (like low testosterone or estrogen)

Sometimes, targeted supplementation or medication under medical supervision can make a dramatic difference. Don't guess; test.

Movement and Morning Light

Movement keeps your energy flowing, like a river that stays clear by constantly moving. There's special power in moving during the transition moments of the day, especially at sunrise. Morning sunlight is a free energy boost, regulating your circadian rhythm and triggering the production of energizing hormones.

Many athletes sit inside an office, behind a desk, most of the day. When your energy feels stagnant, step outside for a walk. Spend some time outside in motion, even if it's gentle. It's not just exercise. It's a practice that can shift your entire energy state for the rest of the day.

Managing Mental Energy

One of the biggest energy drains in modern life isn't physical. It's the constant flood of digital information hitting our minds. Think of your mental energy like a daily allowance. Every notification, scroll and click withdraws from this account.

Try these practices:

- Keep your phone off for the first hour of the day
- Schedule specific times for email and social media rather than constant checking

- Turn off unnecessary notifications on your devices
- Create deliberate periods of information fasting by setting aside one day weekly as a "mental cleanse" with minimal information intake

Many runners report feeling mentally sharper and more energized when they reduce their digital consumption. Their training improves, not just because they have more time but, because they have more mental energy to invest in their running.

Recovery and Downtime

Hard training needs to be balanced with proper recovery. Find something that feels good, that you enjoy doing. Here are some recovery strategies I enjoy:

- 15-minute Epsom salt bath while listening to music
- 30-minute nap, or just resting on the bed
- 30-minute infrared sauna session at 150° F
- 2–3-minute cold plunge at 50° F
- 5-minute breathing exercise (4-7-8 pattern or 4-4 box breathing)
- 20-minute guided meditation session

Watch for signs that indicate you need more recovery: waking up feeling unrefreshed, unusual irritability, decreased motivation, persistent muscle soreness and energy crashes during the day.

Social Energy Management

The people around you can either drain or boost your energy. Every Tuesday night for the past five years, I've met with my close friends Jozef and Duc at my house. We run, hit the sauna, take an ice bath plunge and share dinner together. These evenings consistently leave me feeling energized and restored, no matter how tired I might have been before.

This kind of regular, quality social time isn't just enjoyable; it's essential for maintaining high energy levels. Sometimes, the most powerful energy-management tool is simply saying no to commitments that don't serve your well-being.

Next Steps

1. Set a consistent bedtime for the next week
2. Plan tomorrow's meals today
3. Schedule a blood test if you haven't had one in the past year
4. Turn off notifications on your phone for nonessential apps
5. Book time with someone who energizes you

> **REMEMBER:** Your energy state is largely within your control. Each day presents multiple opportunities to make choices that either enhance or deplete your energy. Choose wisely and watch how it transforms your running and your life.

Chapter Summary

- Your energy multiplies when you optimize sleep, nutrition and stress management together. Small improvements in each area create exponential gains in performance.
- Prioritize 7–9 hours of quality sleep as your most powerful training tool, and manage digital consumption to preserve mental energy throughout the day.
- Use morning light exposure, proper hydration and whole foods to create sustainable energy that supports both training and recovery.

8
The Power of Journaling

A running journal can be one of your most powerful tools for improvement. It's not just about tracking miles; it's about understanding yourself as a runner, and as a person.

Most mornings before my run, I grab my journal and write down three things: how I slept, how my body and mind feel, and what I want to achieve today. This simple practice has transformed not just my running but my entire approach to training.

Why Journal? The Benefits Run Deep

Mental Clarity and Self-Awareness

Running often reveals mental blocks and presents opportunities for breakthroughs. I've found that some of my biggest running insights came not during the run itself but during my post-run journaling session.

Elite mountain runner Kilian Jornet says, "Journaling helps you look back on why things are happening and how they are happening. Memory is often unreliable."

Tracking Progress (Beyond the Numbers)

Sure, your watch can tell you pace, distance and heart rate. But can it tell you why Tuesday's tempo run felt effortless while Saturday's long run was a struggle? Your journal can.

Through consistent journaling I noticed that my best long runs consistently came after days when I'd gotten at least 7.5 hours of sleep and hadn't looked at my phone first thing in the morning. This kind of insight doesn't come from Strava.

Goal Setting and Achievement

World record holder Eliud Kipchoge emphasizes that "improvement goes hand in hand with dedication." Writing down your goals makes them real. The simple act of putting a goal on paper changes how I think about it. It becomes less of a wish and more of a commitment.

Injury Prevention and Stress Management

Your journal can be an early warning system. By tracking how your body feels, you might notice patterns that predict injury before it happens.

I once avoided what could have been a serious Achilles issue because my journal entries showed increasing discomfort after speed sessions—something I might have overlooked if I hadn't been writing it down.

A Simple Running Journal Template

Pre-Run:

- Date/Time:
- Sleep quality (1–10):
- Energy level (1–10):
- Mood:
- Physical niggles:
- Today's goal:
- Any other thoughts:

Post-Run:

- Distance/Time:
- Route:
- How it felt (1–10):
- One thing that worked well:
- One thing to improve:
- Recovery plan:
- Any other thoughts:

Take two minutes before and after your run to complete this. The consistency will reveal patterns you'd never otherwise notice.

Common Pitfalls to Avoid

1. Inconsistency

The biggest mistake I see runners make is journaling sporadically. You don't need to write essays, but consistent brief entries are crucial for spotting patterns. It only takes a few minutes to do. Set a specific time for journaling. I do it during my morning tea and immediately post-run.

2. Numbers-Only Focus

While metrics matter, don't forget the qualitative aspects. How did the run feel? What were you thinking about? I've had "slow" runs that felt amazing and "fast" runs that left me depleted. Your journal should capture these nuances.

3. Not Reviewing

A journal isn't just for writing; it's for learning. I schedule monthly review sessions where I look back through my entries. These reviews have led to some of my biggest training breakthroughs.

Monthly Journal Review Questions:

- What patterns do I notice in my best runs?
- Is there a connection between my sleep quality and running performance?
- Are there any early warning signs of potential injuries?
- Which types of workouts leave me feeling most energized/depleted?
- How has my easy pace changed at the same heart rate?

Next Steps

1. **Keep It Simple:** Start with just three questions after each run:
    - How did I feel?
    - What went well?
    - What could be better?
2. **Make It Convenient:** Keep your journal where you'll see it. I keep mine on my kitchen counter because I walk past it before every run.

3. **Be Honest:** Your journal is for you. No one else needs to see it. The more honest you are, the more valuable the insights will be.
4. **Review Regularly:** Set aside time each month to look back through your entries. You'll be amazed at the patterns you discover.

Digital vs. Physical Journaling

While I prefer a physical journal, many runners use digital options:

- Notes apps on your phone
- Running-specific apps with journaling features
- Voice memo recordings (perfect for immediate post-run thoughts)
- Specialized journaling apps

The best journal is the one you'll actually use consistently.

To help you get started, I've created a simple, proven journal template you can download for free at florisgierman.com/PB-journal.
It's the same one I use daily to stay consistent and reflect on my training. Prefer something you can hold in your hands? A printed (published) version is also available there, perfect to keep on your kitchen counter or toss in your running bag.

Whether you're just getting into journaling or looking to level up your current practice, this tool will help you uncover patterns, track progress and stay on course.

Journaling is one of the most powerful habits my podcast guests have shared over the years. Start small, stay consistent and watch how this simple daily act can transform your running, your health and your life. Your future self will thank you.

Chapter Summary

- Track how you feel before and after runs, along with sleep quality and energy levels, to spot patterns that reveal what truly drives your best performances.
- Monthly journal reviews help you identify early warning signs of injury and understand the real reasons behind breakthrough runs.
- Simple pre- and post-run templates provide more valuable insights than complex data tracking. Consistency matters more than perfection.

9
Run Faster by Relaxing

When I first started running, I thought improvement meant pushing harder on every single run. My mindset was simple: More effort equals better results. For years, this constant pushing left me frustrated, exhausted and frequently injured. Eventually, I learned that to run faster, I actually had to learn how to relax more.

The Hidden Cost of Constant Tension

Many runners, myself included, often make the mistake of thinking that more stress leads directly to better performance. Hard workouts can be helpful for improvement, but too much physical or mental stress without proper recovery quickly becomes counterproductive.

I coached a runner named Mark who should have been crushing his marathon goals. His training was consistent, his nutrition dialed in and his sleep schedule solid. Yet on race day, he'd consistently hit the wall earlier than expected.

During a coaching call, I discovered the issue wasn't his running. It was everything between runs. Mark was in constant stress mode: checking emails first thing in the morning, working through breaks, mentally rehearsing presentations during easy runs and falling asleep with his phone after answering "one more" message.

His body never had a chance to shift out of its stress response. As Dr. Phil Maffetone puts it, "Stress affects our brain, which then impairs fat burning." When stress levels are chronically elevated, your body can't perform optimally, no matter how fit you are.

The 30-Second Tension Check

This quick scan can save tremendous energy over longer distances. During your next run, check in with yourself occasionally to scan for tension:

1. **Face:** Are you clenching your jaw or furrowing your brow? Soften your facial expression.
2. **Shoulders:** Are they hunched toward your ears? Let them drop away from your ears.
3. **Hands:** Are you making tight fists? Imagine holding a potato chip without crushing it.
4. **Breathing:** Is it shallow and rapid? Take three deep belly breaths.
5. **Overall posture:** Are you leaning forward or backward? Align your head over your shoulders.

Why Relaxing Helps You Run Faster

I ran the Tokyo Marathon aiming for a sub-3-hour finish. By mile 22 (35 km), my mind was spiraling into negativity and tension started to tighten my body. Instead of trying harder, I focused on relaxing, breathing more deeply, lowering my shoulders, softening my stride and forcing myself to smile.

The tension disappeared. My energy returned. I crossed the finish in 2:59, feeling lighter than I had in previous races.

This experience taught me that letting go doesn't mean losing control. It means finding flow. This applies for runs and races of all distances, not just marathons. The same principle also applies beyond running. When you resist stress, it compounds. When you learn to release it, everything moves with less effort.

Physical Relaxation for Better Running

As movement specialist Lawrence van Lingen explains, "Movement should be creative, active self-expression. We see so many people that are reactive, defensive or restricted in their movement. I believe wholly that movement should start from the center and should be a creative act whereby you express yourself."

Many runners unintentionally create tension in their body when runs get tough. This extra tension wastes energy, like driving with the emergency brake on.

Common mistakes that create tension:

- Leaning too far forward (keep your head over your shoulders)
- Fighting between upper and lower body
- Head-forward posture
- Overemphasizing the anterior chain without posterior chain engagement
- Clenched fists or tight arms (let your hands stay loose)

The Power of Unhurried Living

One thing I learned from my conversation with Taylor Knibb is how intentional she is about not rushing through her day. She makes a conscious effort to slow down, stay present and keep her stress levels low. That calm off-the-clock mindset allows her to absorb more training and recover faster.

It really struck a chord because I've often found myself doing the exact opposite: rushing out the door, running late to a meeting or school drop-off, already tense before the day's even started. Building in a buffer, just a few extra minutes here and there, has helped reduce that frantic energy. It's not always easy when real life gets messy, but even being aware of it makes a difference. That awareness can be the first step toward more calm, more flow and better running.

Case Study — Maria Lurenda Westergaard: From Anxiety to Personal Best at Any Age

Maria Lurenda Westergaard is redefining what it means to improve as an athlete, even as a self-described "back-of-the-pack runner." Her running journey began in 2013 after witnessing the aftermath of the Boston Marathon bombing, when anxiety threatened to limit her travels and experiences.

"I was nervous; I didn't want to be outside for too long," Maria recalls. "If this happened every time I travel, I would be missing out on a lot of things. If you experience anxiety, the best way to get it out of your system is to do exactly what you are afraid of."

Maria's first attempts at running were humble: alone on a treadmill in her apartment building's basement, embarrassed by her pace of 16 minutes per mile (10 min/km). As a doctor with no athletic background, she approached running with academic rigor, researching everything she could about the sport while gradually building confidence.

Since joining our Personal Best Program, Maria has transformed her approach by tracking four key pillars: stress management, sleep, nutrition and strength training. The results have been incredible. In 2021, she was walking at 19:19 minutes per mile (12:00 per km) with a heart rate of 140. Two years later, she could run at 12:52 minutes per mile (8:00 per km) with a heart rate of 130.

"If I compare how fast I run at a certain heart rate looking at just one week or four weeks, it seems like nothing is happening," Maria explains. "But if I compare my Strava graphs now to two years ago, you can see there's this big change."

Maria's discipline and holistic approach led to a breakthrough at the Berlin Half-Marathon, where despite an emergency hotel evacuation the night before and unexpected allergies, she achieved a personal best of 2:30:14, improving a time she had set 11 years earlier when she was 42.

Using strategies, such as nasal breathing, mindful nutrition and mental techniques, Maria has learned to thrive in challenging circumstances. "Nothing about training, traveling and running events will be perfect," she says. "The goal is to be comfortable in the discomfort."

With a continuous glucose monitor, Maria has also discovered how to manage her prediabetic condition through running, turning potential health challenges into strengths. She's completed multiple half-marathons and marathons across Europe, including Copenhagen, Berlin, Paris, Florence and Athens, always finishing with a smile regardless of her finish time and despite being at the back of the pack.

Her ultimate goal? To run the Boston Marathon when she's 80, returning to where her journey began, but this time as a competitor rather than an observer. This 35-year plan keeps her focused on sustainable training and long-term health rather than short-term gains.

"When you think that long-term, you make different kinds of choices," she says. "Running makes challenging life situations easier to handle. This practice, this discipline of showing up and regulating your emotions to finish the run, actually helps in other parts of life."

Through Maria's journey, we see that personal bests aren't just about pace; they're about finding joy in the process, overcoming limitations and using running as a tool to become healthier and happier at any age.

Full Episode:
extramilest.com/69

Finding Your Flow State

The "flow state," or being "in the zone," a state of immersion where movement feels effortless, is where high-performing athletes thrive.

Here's how to access this powerful state:

1. **Create a Pre-Run Ritual:** I often start with a gentle walk and a few calming breaths, signaling my body and mind to relax.
2. **Practice Mindfulness During Runs:** Bring attention to the present moment—to your footsteps on the ground, your breathing pattern, the wind on your face.
3. **Use Visualization:** Picture yourself running smoothly, relaxed and effortlessly strong.
4. **Focus on Rhythm:** Notice the natural rhythm in your breathing and cadence that emerges when you stop forcing and start flowing.

Running as a Moving Meditation

Relaxation doesn't mean slacking. It means allowing your body to find efficiency and your mind to remain calm, even during challenges. For me, this has turned running into a type of meditation. Rather than fixating on pace or splits, I'm fully immersed in the experience of running itself.

During difficult runs, when tension arises, remind yourself: "Relax. Let go." Keep your form fluid. Lower your shoulders, loosen your grip, and breathe deeply.

Getting Rid of What Slows You Down

Many runners think improved performance comes primarily from building more strength. While some strength is beneficial, eliminating what slows you down is far more important. Otherwise, you're training with the brakes on. The most common limiter? Tension.

Watch elite runner Eliud Kipchoge during his sub-2-hour marathon. He's completely fluid and relaxed at an incredible pace. That's flow state running, when your body moves with perfect efficiency and your mind is fully present, creating effortless power.

Next Steps

1. **Begin with Awareness:** During your next run, do a body scan. Notice where you're holding tension.
2. **Practice Relaxed Running:** Set aside one run per week focused solely on staying relaxed. Don't worry about pace or distance.
3. **Create Stress Buffers:** Implement 30-minute screen-free periods before and after runs.
4. **Develop a Pre-Run Ritual:** Find a simple routine that helps you transition into a flow state.
5. **Breathe Intentionally:** Practice rhythmic breathing during easy runs until it becomes natural.

By learning to release tension and run relaxed, you'll find that your training becomes more enjoyable, your performances improve and the rest of your life feels better, too.

Chapter Summary

- Release unnecessary tension in your face, shoulders and hands during runs to immediately improve efficiency and reduce energy waste.
- Transform running from a constant struggle into a meditative flow state by learning to trust your body's natural movement patterns.
- The 30-second tension check can instantly improve your form and help you discover that speed comes from ease, not force.

10
How to Deal with Frustration in Training

Have you ever felt like you're moving in slow motion while everyone else flies past you? Welcome to the reality of low heart rate training! As someone who's guided thousands of runners through this journey, I want to share the challenges you can expect along the way. We'll also discuss how to turn these frustrations into joy.

The Reality Check

Let's get real about what happens to many runners when they start with low heart rate training:

- Your heart rate skyrockets just minutes into your run
- You slow down dramatically, sometimes to a walk (especially on hills!)
- Runners you used to breeze past now overtake you
- Friends ask if you're injured or sick
- You feel embarrassed to post these "slow" runs online
- You wonder if you calculated your heart rate zones incorrectly
- You finish runs feeling like you barely exercised

Sound familiar? You're not alone! Most runners I coach experience this exact same pattern.

What's Really Happening?

Here's what you need to understand: Your current training pace to keep your heart rate low is simply a reflection of your aerobic development right now, not your potential or fitness level.

Even elite athletes have to dramatically slow down when starting with aerobic training. Six-time Ironman World Champion Mark Allen had to slow his training pace by 3:30 minutes per mile (2:10 min/km) when he first adopted this method!

Your body is making profound adaptations:

- Developing more mitochondria in your muscles
- Improving fat-burning efficiency
- Building capillary networks
- Strengthening connective tissues
- Enhancing cellular energy systems

These changes don't happen overnight, but they're the foundation for lasting performance.

The Mental Game

The biggest obstacle isn't physical, it's mental. Your ego doesn't like going slow. It feels like you're moving backward.

Many runners give up in the early months when they don't seem to be making any progress. But progress requires patience, as the chart on the next page shows.

PATIENT VS. IMPATIENT RUNNER JOURNEY

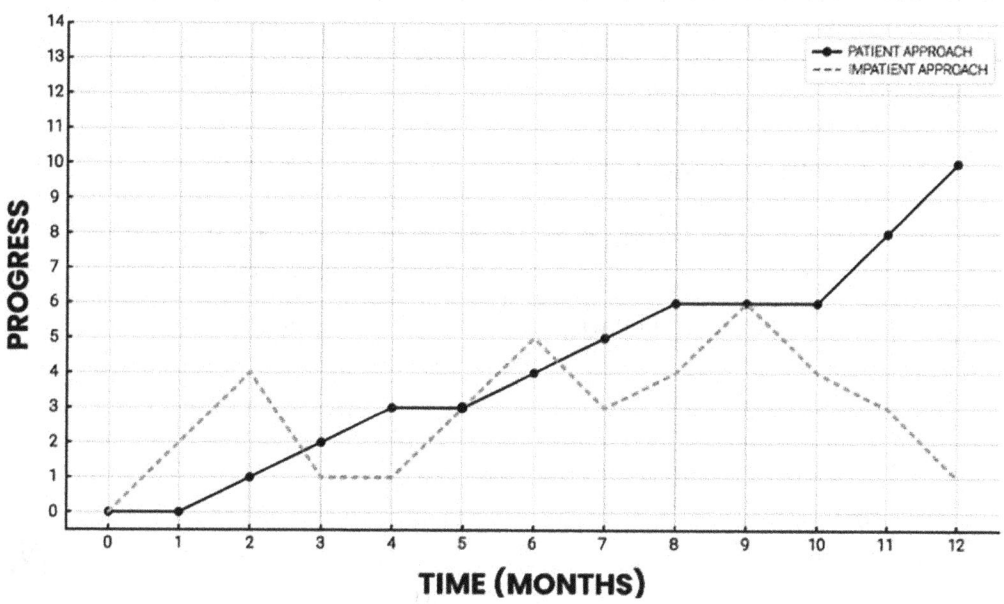

Here's how to shift your mindset:

1. **Reframe your language:** Instead of "problem," think "opportunity." Instead of "struggle," think "journey." Instead of seeing slower runners as "enemies," see them as "teachers."
2. **Give yourself permission:** I'm officially giving you permission to slow down, take walk breaks and finish workouts feeling fresh.
3. **Focus on process, not pace:** Aim to keep your heart rate in the right zone. The pace will take care of itself over time.
4. **Adopt a beginner's mind:** Approach each run with curiosity rather than judgment.
5. **Think long-term:** Ask yourself, "How will I feel about this approach a year from now when I'm running faster with less effort?"

Make It Fun Again

Here are some practical strategies to make low heart rate training more enjoyable:

1. **Turn it into a game**

    - How far can you run before your heart rate alarm goes off?
    - What's the fewest number of alarms you can have in one run?
    - How high up a hill can you get before needing to walk?

2. **Use terrain to your advantage**

    - Downhill sections let you naturally run faster while keeping heart rate low
    - After warming up, try 8-second accelerations with full recovery
    - Find flat routes for building confidence

3. **Try cross-training**

    - Cycling, swimming and hiking can develop aerobic fitness, sometimes with less frustration
    - Mix up activities to keep training fresh

4. **Focus on how you feel**

    - Notice how your recovery improves
    - Pay attention to your energy throughout the day
    - Celebrate finishing runs feeling strong

Troubleshooting When Progress Stalls

If you've been consistent but aren't seeing improvements, consider these common blockers:

- **Stress overload:** Work, family or life stress raises cortisol
- **Poor sleep:** Not enough quality recovery time
- **Nutritional gaps:** Missing key nutrients or experiencing calorie deficits

- **Training inconsistency:** Skipping too many sessions
- **Hidden intensity:** Pushing too hard in "easy" sessions
- **Incorrect training volume:** Either too much or not enough
- **Health issues:** Underlying conditions affecting adaptation

The Question That Matters Most

Are you willing to embrace some temporary frustration for lasting transformation? Are you willing to put aside your ego for better results? Will you trust the process even when immediate feedback isn't visible?

The runners who say yes to these questions are often the ones who ultimately break through to new levels of performance, with more efficiency, fewer injuries and greater enjoyment than ever before.

> **REMEMBER:** You're not going slow forever. You're investing in yourself now to run faster later. Enjoy the process!

Chapter Summary

- The initial slowdown in low heart rate training is temporary and reflects your current fitness, not your potential. Improvements typically appear within 4 to 6 weeks.
- Reframe training frustrations as learning opportunities rather than setbacks, and focus on your individual journey instead of comparing it to others.
- When training feels overwhelming, step back and reconnect with your love for running. Your "why" will carry you through tough moments.

11
Four Drills to Improve Your Running Form

"I just had a massive breakthrough of a run," I said, trying to capture the moment on video with my phone as I talked through the tears. "I pretty much cried the entire time. It was a massive unlocking of emotions and unblocking. I don't know what's going on, but that was the best run of my life."

The Morning Run That Changed Everything

As dawn broke that morning, I headed out to the familiar river ditch near my house. I'd run this path countless times, but today felt different. I set off at a comfortable pace and focused on maintaining a controlled comfortable pace. My form felt effortless: chest open, posterior chain engaged, pelvis rotating smoothly. I just moved with so much more ease than usual, like my body finally understood how to run efficiently.

It was a true breakthrough. Minutes turned into miles as a sense of profound joy came over me. This state of pure flow immersed me in the moment. Tears streamed down my cheeks as emotions welled up inside me.

The transformation came from several movements introduced to me by Lawrence van Lingen, a dear friend and a movement specialist who has helped many endurance athletes overcome injuries and boost their performance.

When I asked Lawrence about these transformative experiences, he explained: "That's what I live for. It's almost a spiritual journey. It's about becoming childlike again, where you are the creator and author of your movement and your life. People become self-aware in terms of movement, like a compartmentalized enlightenment or awakening. You go, 'Ooohhh,' and then everything starts to shift."

The Four Drills That Changed How I Run

1. **The Awesomizer:** Your Hip Mobility Unlock
2. **Flow Rope:** Enhance Your Running Fluidity
3. **Backward Walking:** Prevent Injury and Improve Form
4. **Tire Walking:** Strengthen Your Hips

The Awesomizer: Your Hip Mobility Unlock

Why it works: This drill helps athletes and coaches screen for movement efficiency. You can use it to make your running balanced and symmetrical.

Lawrence explains: "Most people don't realize how much hip mobility affects their running. The Awesomizer helps release tight hips and create fluid movement patterns that translate directly to improved running form."

How to perform (2–4 minutes):

1. Place one foot on a raised surface (about knee height, like a second stair)
2. Rock your hip forward to release the hamstring, repeating to smooth out any tightness or imbalance
3. Add gentle turning movements to open and close your hips while maintaining balance
4. Progress to heel-to-forefoot rocking motions to improve the interaction between foot and hip

Watch the demo at lawrencevanlingen.com/awesomizer

Flow Rope: Enhance Your Running Fluidity

Why it works: "The flow rope teaches you to move from the center out, rather than from the hands in," Lawrence explains. "It helps you develop a rhythm that's grounded in your hips, which is crucial for efficient running."

When I asked Lawrence to explain the concept of the flow rope, he shared: "Think of it like the front of the horse or the back of the horse, or imagine a chimpanzee galloping across the ground. A lot of people are stuck in anterior chain dominant patterns. With the flow rope, you can swing the rope forward, an anterior chain pattern, and swing it in reverse, which lights up the posterior chain pattern."

How to perform (2–4 minutes):

1. Use a rope about 16 mm thick with length equal to the distance from your forearm to the ground.
2. Start by moving the rope in a backward figure-eight pattern, engaging your posterior chain muscles.
3. Add forward movements to alternate between anterior and posterior chain activation.
4. Focus on moving from your hips rather than your hands, allowing your spine and shoulders to respond naturally. Use the rope movement to add fluidity and rhythm to your running.

Lawrence adds: "The pattern is a figure eight. Hips work in a figure-of-eight, and our shoulders work in a figure eight. Restoring that dance or interplay is about getting your shoulders off your hips—one of the primary reasons we use the flow rope. It also decompresses your spine. Once you start animating your spine, your spine becomes fluid."

Watch the demo, or buy a flow rope: lawrencevanlingen.com/flowrope

Backward Walking: Prevent Injury and Improve Form

Why it works: As Lawrence explains, "When you walk backwards, you reverse engineer healthy running form. You get the right extension in your hips, which is what you need for efficient running. Most people, when they run forward, they're collapsing at the hips. Backward walking corrects this by teaching your body how to extend properly."

How to perform (2–3 minutes):

1. Find a clear, safe space and walk backward at a comfortable pace
2. Focus on pushing from your toes through your heel while keeping your chest up and your shoulders relaxed
3. Pay attention to your gait pattern, aiming for opposing arm and leg movement (contralateral movement)
4. Gradually increase distance as you become more comfortable with the movement

"It's about creating a sense of falling forward on a connected leg, which increases efficiency," Lawrence adds. "Backward walking is a way to get familiar with the shape of healthy running."

Watch the demo at lawrencevanlingen.com/backwardswalking

Tire Walking: Strengthen Your Hips

Why it works: This drill strengthens your hips and improves running form by forcing proper hip activation.

"When you pull a tire, you want to focus on keeping your heel down and stepping towards your lead leg," Lawrence explains. "It forces you to use your hips and not your calves or hamstrings. Most people, when they first try this, will find themselves out of balance because they've been relying too much on their anterior chain. Tire pulling helps you shift to using your hips for propulsion."

How to perform (2–4 minutes):

1. Attach a rope about 8 feet long to a tire and step forward toward your lead leg
2. Keep your heel down and focus on using your glutes to move the tire, not just your legs
3. Maintain controlled movement and balance as you practice different directional pulls
4. Gradually increase resistance as your hip strength builds

Watch the demo at lawrencevanlingen.com/tirepull

Why These Drills Work

When I asked Lawrence how often runners should practice these techniques, he emphasized consistency over duration. "Ideally, do these exercises before every run. Start with five minutes of flow rope, five minutes of backward walking and five minutes of tire pulling. Athletes who really commit to this find that it transforms their running. It doesn't take long for your body to adjust, but consistency is key."

For those without access to equipment, Lawrence offers practical alternatives. "For backward walking, you can do it on a treadmill or find a safe, open space like a soccer field. As for the tire, you can get a secondhand tire from a car dealership. They're usually happy to give them away since they have to pay to dispose of them. If you don't have a tire, you can simulate the movement by walking uphill on a treadmill with a slight incline."

5-Minute Quick-Start Routine

When time is limited, here's a simplified routine that combines elements from several drills:

1. **0:00-1:00:** Basic Awesomizer (30 seconds each leg)
2. **1:00-3:00:** Flow rope basic movements (2 minutes)
3. **3:00-5:00:** Backward walking (2 minutes)

Even this short routine, performed consistently, can significantly improve your running mechanics.

You're Never Too Experienced to Learn New Things

I didn't expect that after more than a decade of running I would discover a new approach that would unlock new levels of joy, confidence and flow. The four drills shared in this chapter have changed the way I walk and run, giving me a sense of ease and fluidity I had never previously experienced.

With these tools, you too can transform your running, reduce injuries and find joy in every stride. I hope that you may find trust and let go of fear, and experience a deep sense of connection and joy when you run.

As Lawrence van Lingen says, *"You can't separate motion from emotion. How you move is how you feel. That's why it matters so much the cues you choose and how you perceive running. It massively affects how you feel."*

Embrace these techniques and may your running journey be filled with newfound pleasure and fulfillment.

Chapter Summary

- The Awesomizer and backward walking restore natural hip extension and teach your body the proper movement patterns that modern lifestyle habits have disrupted.
- Flow rope work creates fluidity between upper and lower body while engaging the posterior chain muscles often underused in traditional running.
- Practice these drills consistently before runs to build lasting form improvements that make running feel easier and more efficient.

12
How to Run a Personal Best on Race Day

Achieving a personal best (PB) on race day isn't about luck. It's often the result of months or years of structured training, smart preparation and mental resilience. Whether you're racing a 5K, marathon or ultramarathon, success comes down to four key elements: pacing, fueling, hydration and mindset. This chapter breaks down race day strategies used by me, runners I've coached and guests on my *Extramilest Show*.

Start Smart, Finish Strong

Pacing is crucial for racing success. The most common mistake runners make is starting too fast, a pattern that repeats across all distances. Race day excitement and fresh legs can tempt you to surge early, but I often remind our athletes: "If you shave one minute off in the first few miles, it could cost you five minutes or more later if you start cramping or hitting the wall."

Your pacing strategy should vary by distance:

- **5K & 10K:** Start controlled and build your effort gradually. Avoid the temptation to sprint from the gun. Many beginners burn out within the first mile by starting at an unsustainable pace.
- **Half-Marathon:** Find your sustainable rhythm early and hold it.
- **Marathon:** Learn to hold back. The real race doesn't begin until the 20-mile (32-km) mark. Everything before that is just a long warm-up.

- **Ultramarathon:** Focus on consistent effort rather than pace because energy conservation is more important. Strategic walk breaks early on can make a big difference here.

Remember that even in shorter races, where you can push harder, starting too aggressively is a common reason for missed personal bests. Stay patient and trust your training.

Intensity Discipline on Race Day

In some of my first races, I started too fast and hit the wall big time. Some of these blowups were so miserable I thought I was going to die. But they taught me a lesson about intensity discipline, learning to hold back and avoiding the same mistakes again.

During my Boston Marathon, I watched hundreds of excited runners fly past me in those early miles. By mile 20 (32 km), I was passing them one by one because I'd stayed disciplined with my pacing from the start, finishing in my personal best time of 2 hours, 44 minutes.

Fueling for Success

Your nutrition strategy should be well practiced in training. Never experiment on race day. As Andy Blow notes on *The Extramilest Show* #64, "Many runners assume they're fueling enough, but when we analyze their intake, they're often under-consuming calories and carbs."

Fueling needs by distance:

- **5K & 10K:** No fuel needed during the race; focus on pre-race nutrition
- **Half-Marathon:** Some runners perform well without mid-race fueling, but taking in 30–60 g carbs per hour can help maintain energy
- **Marathon:** Aim for 60–90 g of carbs per hour
- **Ultras:** Combine liquid carbs, gels and real food to change things up and to prevent energy crashes

Train your gut by progressively increasing carb intake during training sessions. This helps your body adapt to processing nutrition while running, reducing the risk of GI issues on race day.

For marathons and ultras, I have trained my way up to 90 grams of carbs per hour (I take 30 g carbs every 20 minutes, usually from gels); however, experimenting in training is key.

Smart Hydration Strategy

As hydration expert Andy Blow emphasizes, "Dehydration and overhydration both hurt performance. A strategic hydration plan, based on sweat rate, helps you avoid both pitfalls."

Key hydration principles:

- Races under 2 hours: minimal hydration needed unless it's hot
- Longer races: plan electrolyte intake alongside fluids
- Hot conditions or heavy sweater: consider preloading with electrolytes
- High sweat rate: may need 500–1,500 mg sodium per hour

Avoid the common mistake of drinking too much plain water without electrolytes, which can lead to hyponatremia in longer events.

Race Week Timeline

- Many runners sabotage their races with excessive training during taper week. The goal is fresh legs and a rested body at the starting line. Consistently reduce both volume and intensity as race day approaches.
- Gradually increase carbohydrate intake in the days before your race without overdoing it; no need for extreme carbo-loading that leaves you feeling bloated or uncomfortable.
- A short, easy 15–30 minute shakeout run the day before can maintain neuromuscular readiness without depleting energy stores.
- Stick with proven nutrition; use the same dinner and breakfast that worked well during your training runs. Race week is never the time to experiment with new foods or timing.

Build Mental Resilience

Racing tests your mental strength as much as your physical capabilities. Every runner faces moments when their body and mind urge them to stop. The key to breakthrough performances lies in preparing for these challenges before they arise.

Race Day Mental Techniques:

- **Chunking:** Break the race into smaller segments (aid station to aid station)
- **Mantras:** Prepare two or three short phrases to repeat when things get tough
- **Form focus:** When discomfort increases, focus on running form instead
- **Engagement:** High-five spectators, thank volunteers
- **Smiling:** Deliberately smiling, even when it's hard, can reduce perceived effort

Case Study: Duc Tran's Sub 3-Hour Marathon Journey

For Duc Tran, running marathons was a journey marked by extremes. Coming from a CrossFit and triathlon background, Duc carried the intense "no pain, no gain" mindset into his running, which repeatedly landed him in the medical tent after races.

"I did Boston 2018, and that year the weather was just fantastic, near freezing temperatures, raining, a lot of wind," Duc recalls with a hint of sarcasm. "I went to the medical tent. I couldn't stop shaking."

Despite completing multiple Ironmans and marathons with impressive times, Duc couldn't break the elusive sub-3-hour barrier. At 44 years old, the Irvine, California, runner and father of two knew something had to change.

"My first half-marathon was brutal," Duc says. "I cramped so severely my friend had to carry me back to the car. I didn't learn my lesson right away."

His Training Transformation

Inspired by *The Extramilest Show*, Duc reached out to me about low heart rate training. His transition to lowering his training intensity wasn't easy.

"It was a tough pill to swallow. My easy pace used to be around 7:30 to 8:30 per mile (4:40 to 5:17 per km). Now, I had to run slower than 9-minute miles (5:36 km) just to stay within my heart rate zone," Duc admits. "It's a blow to the ego, but you have to change your mindset and embrace the principle."

After three months of consistent base building at his heart rate of around 141 bpm, the magic started happening. His pace at the same effort improved from around 8:30 per mile to 7:20 (5:17 to 4:33 per km).

"Once the aerobic system gets built, it can absorb the higher intensity training, and that's when you really start to see the benefits. You're running faster at the same effort level."

Race Day Success

When the Boston Marathon was postponed during the pandemic, Duc made the decision to continue training and attempt a solo sub-3-hour marathon on the original race date. I joined him on a bike for the first 20 miles (32 km) and ran the last 6 miles (10 km) with him.

"My goal was simply to break three hours," Duc recalls. "But around mile 20 (32 km), instead of hitting the wall, I felt fantastic. I had enough left to pick up the pace."

He finished in an outstanding 2:56:12, crushing his goal by nearly 4 minutes. Even more remarkable was his recovery.

"Usually, I'm limping for a week and can't walk down stairs. This time, I was ready to run again just a day and a half later."

The Bigger Lesson

While Duc celebrates his faster times, he emphasizes the broader benefits of his new training approach.

Duc has found sustainable joy in running: "I don't really care about pace anymore. It's pure enjoyment just to run. You become a healthier athlete. You can run every day and feel injury-free."

Since his breakthrough sub-3 marathon, Duc has continued to improve, running an impressive 2:45 at the Ventura Marathon and completing Ironman Cozumel in 9:23. His advice to other runners is simple: Be patient, be consistent and be a good listener to your body. The results, as his journey proves, are well worth the wait.

Full Episode:
extramilest.com/34

Chapter Summary

- Smart pacing is the foundation of breakthrough performances. Start conservatively and build gradually to avoid the devastating slowdown that ruins most race attempts.
- Plan your fueling strategy (60–90 g carbs per hour for marathons) and practice it in training. Race day is never the time to experiment with nutrition.
- Stay present and use mental techniques like chunking the distance and mantras to maintain focus when the race gets tough.

13
What to Do When the Sh*t Hits the Fan

Mike Tyson said it best: "Everyone has a plan until they get punched in the mouth." On race day, the punch could be bad weather, a cramping muscle, a fueling mistake or just hitting the wall hard unexpectedly. You won't always see it coming, but you can control how you respond.

The Runner's Emergency Toolkit

Scenario: Off-Pace Early

- Immediate action: Don't panic or try to "make up time."
- Recalibrate expectations based on current conditions.
- Break the remaining distance into smaller chunks.
- Mental approach: "Today's race is different than planned, but I can still perform my best under these conditions."

Scenario: Upset Stomach

- Immediate action: Slow down your pace. Find a bathroom if necessary.
- Slow your intake of fuel temporarily.
- Switch to more diluted fluids, if possible.
- Mental approach: "This setback costs minutes, not my whole race."

Scenario: Unexpected Cramping

- Immediate action: Gently stretch. Slow down but don't stop completely, if possible.
- Check hydration and electrolytes.
- Try to stay as relaxed as possible.
- Mental approach: "This is temporary, I can work through this."

Step 1: Accept Reality, Then Adapt

When things go south, fighting reality only burns more energy. The faster you accept what's happening, the faster you can adjust.

At the Berlin Marathon, I had one clear goal: Run under 3 hours. But three weeks before the race, I injured my calf and had to stop my training runs. I barely ran in the final weeks leading up to race day and mostly did some cross-training. I knew I wasn't in peak shape, but I still wanted to give it my best shot.

What I've learned is that runners often go through five stages with setbacks: denial, anger, bargaining, depression and acceptance. The longer you stay in those first four negative stages, the more energy you waste. Instead of being stuck in denial or anger about my injury, I skipped straight to acceptance. This allowed me to focus on solutions: resting properly, active recovery, cross-training, getting treatment and adjusting my goals.

Step 2: Stay Calm and Stay in the Moment

When discomfort hits, panic makes it worse. Instead of spiraling, control what you can:

- **Relax your shoulders:** tension wastes energy
- **Slow your breath:** calms your mind and body
- **Shift your mindset:** from "this sucks" to "I can handle this"

In Berlin, I caught myself clenching up. My heart rate spiked, and negative thoughts crept in. I forced myself to smile. It sounds ridiculous, but it worked. Smiling relaxed my body and reset my mindset from "I'm falling apart" to "One step at a time."

At mile 15 (24 km), the crowd's energy gave me a boost. I remember thinking, "If this doesn't give you energy, I don't know what will." When negative thoughts came ("pity party for my left calf"), I quickly overrode them with "Run the moment; enjoy this experience."

Step 3: Shrink the Challenge

When finishing a race feels impossible, make the goal smaller:

- Can't think about the next 10 miles (16 km)? Just get to the next aid station.
- That still feels too big? Just get to the next streetlight.
- Still overwhelmed? Focus on one breath, one step at a time.

By mile 22 (35 km), my pace slowed and my legs felt like bricks. Instead of thinking about the final 4 miles (6 km), I told myself: "Just stay on the blue line, one step at a time." Breaking it down like that kept me moving forward.

Step 4: Control What You Can

You can't control race day weather, unexpected cramps or other runners cutting you off. But you can control:

- Your effort
- Your mindset
- Your fueling and pacing decisions

I couldn't change my calf pain, but I could adjust my expectations, take in extra fuel and focus on running relaxed. That mindset shift saved my race.

At mile 16 (26 km), I took some caffeine as a pick-me-up because I was hitting a rough patch. By mile 20 (32 km), running a 6:53 min/mile pace (4:17 min/km) felt incredibly difficult, but I focused on what I could control: my form, my breathing and my attitude.

Step 5: Reframe Setbacks as Growth

A bad race isn't a failure; it's a lesson. Setbacks force you to adjust, learn and grow. The best runners aren't the ones who never struggle. They're the ones who keep learning and adapting.

Step 6: Draw Strength from Community

Running can feel like a solo sport, but the power of community is real. In my toughest moments, encouragement from others has pulled me through.

At mile 21 (33 km) in Berlin, seeing familiar faces from my Personal Best Program gave me an incredible boost. That brief connection—a cheer, a familiar face, a few words of encouragement—can completely change your mindset when you're suffering.

The Real Path to Success

Progress: Expectation Versus Reality

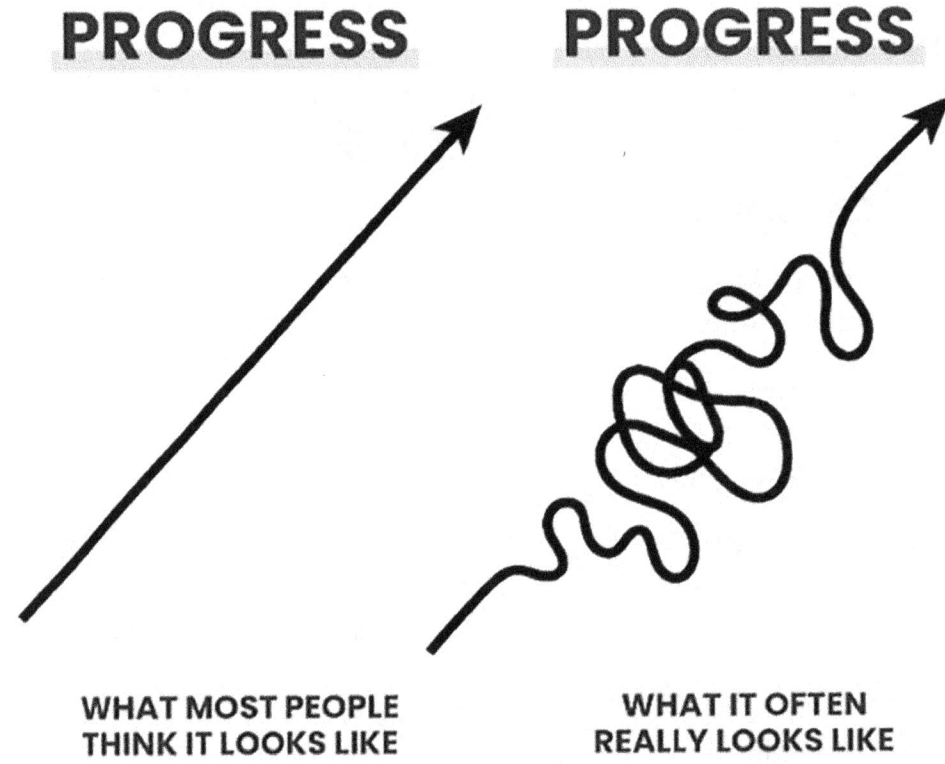

Setbacks don't mean failure. They're part of the journey forward.

Final Thought

The way you handle the hardest moments defines you as a runner and shapes how you'll face future challenges. When the sh*t hits the fan, don't fight it. Accept, adapt, stay present and keep moving.

As I told myself while crossing that finish line in Berlin: "We can do hard things." That lesson extends far beyond running, into your work life, family life and everything else that matters.

Chapter Summary

- Accept reality quickly and adapt to changing conditions rather than fighting what's happening. This conserves energy for finding solutions.
- Break overwhelming challenges into smaller pieces: Focus on reaching the next aid station rather than thinking about the finish line 13 miles away.
- Stay calm using deep breathing, and control what you can (effort, mindset, fueling) while letting go of what you can't (weather, equipment failures).

14
Yes, Older Runners CAN Still Improve

"I'm 51 and finding running harder these days. Can I still improve? Or is my best running behind me?"

This question comes up frequently from recreational runners in their forties, fifties and beyond. The short answer? Absolutely yes, you can still improve as an older runner. Let me share some truth about running as we age.

The "Slow Down" Myth

Many believe your pace inevitably declines after 50, but your body doesn't suddenly stop adapting to training! Older runners can still respond to proper training stimuli. We just need the right approach.

Walter Liniger didn't start low heart rate training until his late sixties. At 69, he completed his first 100K ultramarathon feeling strong throughout. "Stay in the moment," he says. "Take one step after another and see what comes from that."

The key? Consistency over intensity. Walter found his body needed gentler, more patient training to work with his physiology rather than against it.

The Recovery Challenge

As we age, recovery does take longer, but that doesn't mean we can't improve! The solution is smarter training, not less training.

Personal Best Program member Jennifer Kellett is an accomplished marathon runner. After beginning to run seriously in 2015 at age 60, Jennifer has set multiple records, including a personal best of 3:23 at age 69.

"I don't get up and say I have to do this today. I get up and ask how do I feel," says Kellett.

This intuitive approach has allowed her to maintain 60+ mile (100 km) weeks consistently without injuries. Rather than following rigid training schedules, Jennifer listens to her body and adjusts accordingly.

Recovery Strategies for Older Runners:

- Prioritize sleep quality (aim for 7–9 hours).
- Consider adding extra recovery days between hard efforts.
- Use cross-training (swimming, cycling) to maintain fitness while reducing impact.
- Practice active recovery (gentle walking, yoga) rather than complete rest.
- Monitor morning heart rate for signs of incomplete recovery.

The Strength Connection

Studies show age-related performance decline is closely linked to muscle mass loss, which is preventable! After age 30, we naturally lose 3%–5% of muscle mass per decade, but resistance training can dramatically slow or even reverse this process.

Andrea Hudson Baldwin, born in 1959, is a dedicated runner and family nurse practitioner based in Dallas, Texas. Since starting consistent training in 2015, Andrea has achieved personal records across all race distances, with her marathon PR of 3:28:11 set at the Chicago Marathon.

She incorporates strength training twice weekly. When she added consistent resistance work, her times dropped dramatically despite being in her sixties. Just two 20-minute sessions weekly focusing on legs, core and balance can dramatically improve your running economy!

Simple Strength Routine for Older Runners:

- Squats (bodyweight or with light weights)
- Single-leg balancing exercises
- Core work (planks, bird dogs)
- Hip strengthening (clamshells, bridges)
- Upper body maintenance (push-ups, rows)

The Mindset Matters

Perhaps the biggest limit ISN'T physical at all.

Society constantly tells older runners to lower expectations. Phrases like "not bad for your age" or "just finishing is an achievement" can subconsciously limit what we believe is possible.

"Age is not the real barrier that a lot of us think it is," Jennifer Kellett says. The mental freedom of rejecting age limitations allowed her to train with purpose rather than resignation.

Set ambitious goals, ignore the naysayers and surround yourself with positive examples. I've seen countless runners in their fifties, sixties and seventies achieve times they never thought possible, often faster than their younger selves!

Your Long-Game Advantage

Here's what some younger runners don't have: perspective and patience. "Never think about what you have to do, only about what you already did," says Liniger.

This present-focused mindset reduces anxiety, creates enjoyment and leads to consistency, which is the best way to improve at any age.

Your edge: You understand that improvement comes gradually. This patience is your superpower. If you've never done that dream run, you absolutely still can.

Success Stories by Personal Best Program Members That Prove Age Is Just a Number:

- Eric Gustavsen (61 years old) dropped his 10K from 61 minutes to 40:58 and improved his marathon from 3:47 to 3:19.
- Jonathan Pitayanukul (64 years old) improved his 5K from 27:49 to 24:07 and dropped 16 minutes off his marathon time to run 3:54 in just 5 months.
- Ayako Fackenthal (59 years old) went from "relatively sedentary" for 55 years to running her first 50-mile (80-km) ultra in just 3 years. She also improved her marathon by 30 minutes to 4:30 with negative splits.
- John Koontz (47 years old) completed the JFK 50-miler (80 km) with a controlled heart rate below 150 bpm, demonstrating outstanding endurance and disciplined training.

Training Differently, Not Less

The key to continued improvement isn't training less but training smarter. Here's what works for successful older runners:

1. **Build aerobic efficiency:** Low heart rate training becomes even more valuable as we age. Training mostly at an aerobic pace works particularly well for master runners.
2. **Emphasize consistency over heroic workouts:** Some high-intensity running is also important for older runners to optimize health and performance. Don't kill yourself in workouts. Consistency matters most.
3. **Monitor recovery metrics:** Track how you feel. Monitor your morning resting heart rate or heart rate variability. These signals become more important with age.
4. **Make strength non-negotiable:** Even one or two short weekly sessions can make a tremendous difference in running economy and injury prevention.
5. **Address mobility:** Add dynamic movement patterns before runs and gentle stretching afterward to maintain range of motion.

Age brings wisdom if we're willing to apply it to our running. Listen to your body; train smarter not harder, and remember that the best age to be a runner is whatever age you are right now.

The desire to improve doesn't have an expiration date. Whether you're 55, 65 or 75, your next personal best is still out there waiting for you.

Chapter Summary

- Age-related performance decline is largely preventable through consistent training and strength work. Lifestyle factors matter more than chronological age.
- Embrace your advantages in patience and consistency, which make older runners ideally suited for the long-term approach that produces lasting improvements.
- Prioritize recovery and train smarter, not less. Focus on aerobic development and movement quality rather than high-intensity volume.

PART 4
Experts in Conversation

Becoming a stronger, healthier and happier runner isn't just about running more. A lot of factors play a role: nutrition, sleep, stress, recovery, mindset and even how you move. When I became more serious about running in 2013, I had so many questions about how to train smarter and take better care of my body. So I started reaching out to coaches, scientists, health professionals and other experts to learn from the best.

In this section, I've pulled together some of the most helpful conversations I've had with top experts in their fields. You'll hear from Dr. Stephen Seiler on training intensity, Patrick McKeown on breathwork, Dr. Phil Maffetone on holistic endurance training, Dr. Rangan Chatterjee on building better habits and Lawrence van Lingen on running form and movement efficiency.

These are the kinds of insights I wish I had known earlier in my running journey. The more you understand about your body and training, the better choices you can make, not just for running but for your overall health and well-being. I hope these expert conversations help you as much as they've helped me.

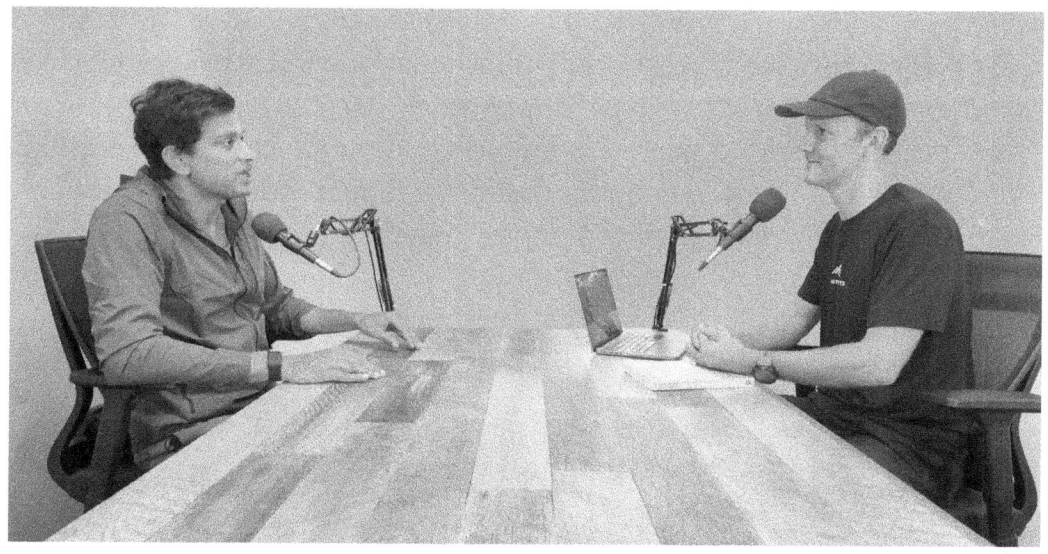

A conversation with Dr. Rangan Chatterjee on how to create healthy habits that last.

Dr. Stephen Seiler on 80/20 Training

"You don't have to go hard every day in training with high-intensity sessions. You're building the cake, but racing is eating. You have to balance that. If you eat the cake too much, then you're going to be in trouble."

Dr. Stephen Seiler is an exercise physiologist, a professor in sport science at the University of Agder in Norway and one of the world's leading minds in the science of cycling. He has authored hundreds of peer-reviewed publications and popular science articles. His identification of the 80/20 rule, a polarized training regimen that sees elite athletes spend 80% of their training at lower intensities and 20% at higher intensities, has become widely accepted among a broad range of elite and endurance athletes. These include cross-country skiers, rowers, cyclists and long-distance runners.

Connect:
x.com/StephenSeiler

Full Episode:
extramilest.com/50

Training Fundamentals

Can you explain the concept of training hierarchy with volume, intensity and overall distribution?

If you haven't done anything, almost anything will make you better as an untrained person over a few months. But if you've only ever measured that initial phase, you miss the point that it stagnates. Different information emerges when you measure highly trained athletes.

When talking about intensity distribution, you scale it down to three zones and five zones. It's been given these different names, like polarized, 80/20 and things like that. The fundamental commonality, the most consistent thing you see, is that most of the best performers, independent of endurance sport, if their event lasts four or five minutes or longer, all the way out to hours and hours, are training fairly similarly. Most of their training intensity is, in physiological terms, below that first lactate turn point. In everyday language, you would say they're training at what, for them, is a fairly easy pace, a talking pace, fairly comfortable. But they're doing it sometimes for a long time.

You don't have to go full speed to get those adaptations. Now, they do some of that high-intensity work also. There's more variability. This is consistently there, but how they manipulate it, whether it's threshold or closer to VO_2 max, varies. The big picture is that humans can't train hard every day. The human will break down. The training process is a yin and yang process. You're trying to use exercise to induce signals that drive protein synthesis, build more mitochondria and so on. But training is also stressful, challenging the body and disturbing homeostasis.

It becomes an optimization problem, not a maximization problem. Maximization doesn't work; it's about finding a rhythm of signal, recovery and adaptation. We're seeing data now that provide mechanistic explanations for why athletes have evolved in that direction.

Does the 80/20 approach work as well for the recreational runner as it does for the elite athlete?

The answer is, in some ways, it works even better for the recreational runner. Here's what I mean. If you're a high-performance athlete pushing the limits, it almost forces you into a certain pattern. You can't train 25 hours a week and go hard every day. But if you're training four or five days a week, say 8 hours a week, you can fall into the temptation to go medium-hard every day.

Recreational athletes often make the mistake of spending time in that yellow zone, a no man's land that is not slow enough, not hard enough. It's easy to fall into that trap, especially with platforms like Zwift, where you start chasing other riders. The most common training mistake age groupers make is this regression towards the mean, which is medium-hard intensity, fairly short workouts, repetitive and monotonous loads. I can't even count how many messages I've received from people who say they've finally learned how to ease up on their easy days and have seen significant improvements. It's anecdotal, but I've had so much of it from regular folks who have experienced new performance records in their fifties.

Intensity and Stress Management

We've talked about the easy part, but what about the hard part? Can you talk about not going too hard on the hard days?

You don't have to go hard every day in training with high-intensity sessions. You're building the cake, but racing is eating. You have to balance that. If you eat the cake too much, then you're going to be in trouble. The term "polarized training" might be misleading because it implies that easy is easy and hard is even harder, which isn't always the case.

Training is about finding a sustainable pattern of loading. My daughter exemplifies this. When I told her to do three or four times 8 minutes on the treadmill, she would push herself too hard, making every interval session a test of her toughness.

Eventually, I had to put the brakes on her and say "You're blowing yourself up and not recovering fast enough." I had to specify a heart rate limit, and once she adhered to that, everything got better. She started setting personal records and fell into a rhythm. Kipchoge, for example, talks about wanting to finish a workout still smiling, so he can train the next day. It's about finding a balance between pushing yourself and not going too deep into the well.

How does this philosophy apply to recreational runners, especially when it comes to stress management?

Stress is a significant factor. Athletes often feel overwhelmed, and it's crucial to recognize when stress levels are high and adjust training accordingly. Sometimes, it's better to push out races and focus on maintenance mode for overall health and relaxation rather than putting the pedal to the metal.

There have been studies showing that scholarship athletes in the United States are less responsive to training during exam periods due to stress. The body doesn't differentiate the source of stress, whether it's from an exam, a breakup or an interval session. It's all the same bucket, and when the bucket is full, performance suffers.

Technology and Training Success

What are your thoughts on the impact of modern technology, like heart rate monitors and bio-tracking tools, on training?

Modern technology has come a long way, from bulky heart rate monitors to sleek devices like the heart rate armbands. These tools provide valuable data, but the key is to use them to inform decisions, not to let them dictate your training.

One area I'm particularly interested in is breathing. It's often overlooked, but it's a vital sign that can provide insight into how hard you're working. For example, breathing frequency tracks better with the reality of your effort in interval sessions than heart rate does. We're looking into how breathing can be used as an intensity scale and help athletes better manage their training.

It's important to remember that many world-class athletes achieve success without relying on all this tech. The simplicity of listening to your body and focusing on the fundamentals should never be underestimated.

Favorite Takeaways from Our YouTube Community

@timshearn8203 – "Training is building the cake, racing is eating it." Thanks for another great video, Floris.

@bobdepradines1773 – The light-bulb moment for me was "get healthy first then train, otherwise the best case scenario is nothing happens!"

@Landauian – Favorite quote: "It becomes an optimization problem. It's not a maximization problem." This is key for me to remember. More miles aren't better if they're chipping away at my ability to adapt to the training.

@IDKDCA – "Your muscles' cells aren't that sophisticated … get some high-intensity work in … approximations end up being close enough often"—the absolute sports science GOAT—love it.

@richardverrier7970 – "Great endurance athletes have intensity discipline." As a recreational runner, I need to park my ego aside. "Training is about finding a sustainable pattern of loading. Learn how to ease up on easy days and figure out what easy means." I realize my runs are too often in the so-called no man's land (Z3), not slow enough, not hard enough.

Dr. Rangan Chatterjee on Healthy Habits

"While making a hot drink, why not do 10 squats, 10 lunges on each leg and 10 calf raises? I promise you, if you do that every morning for 7 days, or even better, a month, your legs will become significantly stronger, and you'll adapt very quickly."

Dr. Rangan Chatterjee is a runner, renowned doctor, author and podcast host of *Feel Better, Live More*. He is regarded as one of the most influential doctors in the UK. A practicing GP for over two decades, he inspires sustainable lifestyle changes through his #1 health podcast on Apple Podcasts in the UK, bestselling books and his TED talk, "How to Make Diseases Disappear," which has been viewed almost 6 million times.

Connect:
instagram.com/drchatterjee

Full Episode:
extramilest.com/90

Small Steps for Lasting Change

Many runners make big lifestyle changes all at once. You emphasize small steps instead. Why does this approach work better?

A huge part of my job is helping people make changes in their lives that actually last. We can all make changes for a few weeks, maybe a few months, but they often don't stick. There are a few key principles that work most of the time, backed by scientific evidence.

The first rule is to make it easy. If a behavior is difficult, you'll do it when motivation is high, but the moment it drops, you won't stick with it. This is why New Year's resolutions often fail.

The second rule is attaching a new behavior to an existing habit. Everything we do in life is triggered by something. The best trigger is sticking a new behavior onto something you already do. For example, I do a 5-minute strength workout every morning while waiting for my coffee to brew. It's easy, automatic, and has become part of my routine. Small, consistent actions accumulate over time.

The third rule is creating an environment that supports your behavior. I keep a kettlebell and a dumbbell in my kitchen, making it easy to pick them up daily. If I stored them away, I'd never use them. This principle applies to everything. My kids see me lifting weights in the kitchen, so they pick them up too. The environment we create shapes our behaviors and those of the people around us.

These small steps might seem insignificant, but they compound into something powerful. If you make it easy, attach it to an existing habit, and set up your environment for success, the behavior becomes automatic. The same principles apply to running, strength training, nutrition, anything you want to incorporate into your life.

Many runners chase faster times, sometimes at the expense of enjoying the process. How can runners set themselves up for success without losing the joy of running?

For much of my life, I was driven by external validation. My parents, immigrants from India to the UK, believed excelling in school would protect me from struggles they faced. As a child, I interpreted their expectations as needing to achieve to be loved. This shaped my drive to always chase success. When I got into running, I was obsessed with beating my times, but eventually, I had to ask myself: Why? Was I running for the right reasons, or was I still chasing external approval?

Everything in life has an upside and a downside. Tracking times and striving for improvement can be motivating, but constantly chasing a "perfect race" can be exhausting. We are never the same runner on any given day. Sleep, stress, weather and countless factors play a role. I've met many runners who define themselves by their personal bests, and when they can't hit those numbers anymore, their relationship with the sport suffers. Some even stop running altogether because they can't accept slowing down.

I would encourage runners to ask: Why am I so focused on this goal? If breaking 20 minutes in a 5K is about proving your worth, the joy will be fleeting. But if it's about challenging yourself in a healthy way, then it can be a great motivator.

I've experimented with running without a watch for six months. I still love data, but I wanted to see if I could tune in to my body without relying on a device. This process has been eye-opening. I'm learning to feel my effort levels rather than letting a screen dictate my run. The real power of technology is when it enhances our ability to listen to ourselves, not when it replaces our own intuition.

Purpose over Performance

Many runners unknowingly push too hard, spending most of their training runs in Zone 3 or 4 when they think they're taking it easy. When they finally slow down, it's eye-opening. You've gone through a period of mostly low heart rate training. What has that process taught you?

Chapter 1 of my book is called "Trust Yourself," and it's my favorite chapter. I've spent 23 years as a doctor helping people change behaviors, and one thing I've learned is that no single approach works for everyone. We all have different stress levels, beliefs and backgrounds, which means the best approach is personal.

I get messages all the time from people confused by conflicting expert advice, with one saying a low-carb diet is best and another saying endurance athletes need high carbs. Instead of asking, Which expert should I trust?, the better question is Why do I no longer trust myself? Information is valuable, but the real power comes from self-experimentation. Try an approach for four weeks. Observe how you feel: your energy, recovery, sleep, mood. Then, try another. Through experience, you'll learn what works for you at that moment in time.

Running is a perfect tool for developing self-awareness if we let it. When we pay attention during our runs, we start to understand ourselves better. How do we react to discomfort? Can we tune in to effort without relying on data? These are skills that not only improve running but carry over into life.

Your Body Can Tell You More than Your Devices

Wearables sometimes give data that doesn't match how we feel. How do you handle this disconnect?

I once asked Eliud Kipchoge if he checks his Oura data before a race. His answer? "Never." It's irrelevant on race morning. In training, it helps, but when it's time to perform, he trusts his body. Research shows that belief about sleep can impact performance. One study told people who slept five hours that they had actually slept eight, and their energy levels improved just from that belief.

Wearables can be useful, but some runners become dependent on the data, letting it dictate their training instead of listening to their body. Technology is great when it enhances awareness, but the real goal should be learning to trust your own signals.

Why do athletes push beyond their limits and overtrain, despite knowing the importance of gradual progression and proper recovery?

It's human nature. We know better, yet we push ourselves too hard. The key is to recognize these moments and adjust before injuries force us to stop.

One of the biggest things I learned from Eliud Kipchoge is how rarely he gets injured, because he listens to his body. If something starts to feel off, he doesn't ignore it. He asks: Is there an imbalance? Do we need to adjust?

Many recreational runners brush off small aches. They finish a run thinking that their Achilles is a little sore, but instead of addressing it, they ice it, rest and keep going. The problem? If you feel it at a 5K, you'll definitely feel it at a 10K or a marathon. These signals don't disappear on their own.

Kipchoge doesn't ignore a niggle. Neither should you.

Start Small, Start Smart

What advice would you give to someone just starting their running journey?

I passionately believe that humans are born to run. But our modern lifestyles aren't exactly designed to support that. I believe the reason so many people get injured when they start running isn't because running is inherently bad for the body. It's because we've developed imbalances from the way we live: sitting all day, hunching over our phones—all sorts of modern habits.

I go for 10-minute runs. I've noticed there's this black-and-white thinking in fitness. If it's not a long session, what's the point? No, go for a 10-minute run. Do that regularly, and you'll build up quickly. In fact, in some ways, it's better because you're adapting gradually, reducing strain on your body.

I always do a 10-minute walking warm-up first. Helen Hall, who I've worked with for five years, really helped me see that the body needs to be primed before running. The blood needs to be diverted to the extremities. I've had injuries in the past that I think could have been prevented with proper warm-ups. I've also become a huge fan of walking warm-downs.

If I have one hour for a run, I now see that 40 minutes of running plus a 10-minute warm-up and 10-minute warm-down is much better than a straight 60-minute run. It takes time to adopt that mindset because the Western mentality is to maximize every minute. But I've realized I get the most out of my run when I take that extra time to warm up and cool down.

Running is a gift. If you take care of yourself, it will keep giving. I want to be running when I'm 70, 80, 90. That's the long game. If you're dealing with pain, don't assume you have to stop running. Have you tried adjusting your diet? Your form? Your recovery? I've seen so many people make small changes like cutting out processed foods or improving their movement, and their pain disappears. Everything is connected: the way we train, eat, sleep, recover, manage stress.

Hearing Your Own Thoughts

Can you tell me more about why you take a summer break from social media, and what you've learned from it?

I've recorded four conversations with Gabor Maté on my podcast, and for our most recent one, I wanted to approach it differently. I decided to frame it around *The Top Five Regrets of the Dying*, and that episode became the most downloaded one of the year.

There is a viral clip online from that conversation where Gabor reflects on his own regrets. Despite all his success with the bestsellers and the global recognition, he admitted he wouldn't live his life the same way if he could do it again. The cost was too high. He worked too much, wasn't as present with his family as he wanted to be and forgot to play.

That conversation resonated deeply with me because I've been thinking about these ideas for years, especially since my dad passed away in 2013. He worked incredibly hard, doing full-time shifts plus four nights a week for 30 years, only sleeping three nights a week. Of course, he got sick. He had dreams for retirement, but he never got to live them. That made me question my own choices. Am I waiting for some future moment to start living?

That's why I take summers off. Four weeks, sometimes six. I travel with my wife and kids, we have adventures, and I delete social media from my phone. Every year, I'm reminded of how much external noise influences my thinking. We absorb so many opinions without realizing it. When I step away, I start to hear my own thoughts again. What do I actually believe? Is my life aligned with what matters most to me?

And that, to me, is priceless.

What advice would you give to runners looking to become stronger, healthier and happier in their training and their everyday lives?

Awareness alone doesn't lead to change. Inspiration without action won't get you anywhere. If there was one thing in this conversation that stuck with you, don't just forget about it and move on with your day. Actually take a moment and ask yourself how you are going to address that.

You don't have to change everything overnight. Maybe you know you're not doing enough strength training, but getting to the gym twice a week feels unrealistic. Okay, maybe you start with a 5-minute workout every morning while your coffee is brewing.

Just remember, no single approach works for everyone. Take what we've discussed, filter it through your own life, and ask, Is this right for me? If it is, take action. If it's not, let it go.

Favorite Takeaways from Our YouTube Community

@toriganaku – I AM 80 years old and still running and intend to do so for many years to come. I just purchased the new Lonely Planet book titled *Epic Runs in North America*, and I'm looking forward to doing some. My favorite takeaway is to lop 20 minutes off my hour-long run for a 10-minute walking warm-up and a 10-minute walking cooldown. Lovely interview. Thank you.

@jackies6274 – The biggest takeaway for me is that if I keep looking after myself, the results will come. I've been so focused on trying to speed up those results that I've neglected other important factors like rest and nutrition, thinking they are of lesser importance, and it has slowly impacted my consistency. I needed to hear this!

@thadstuart8544 – This was a fascinating discussion. My favorite takeaway was to evaluate if I'm pursuing running times and finishing running events for external validation. I believe I am guilty of this. I intend to pursue "the long game" as he described it, and focus more on the internal benefits of running like stress relief, overall life balance, etc. Thanks for sharing this wonderful guest!

@runningwoman7207 – Loved this video! Learned so much! Best takeaway for me … would be the idea of 5 min in the morning to do squats, heel raises, etc., while making coffee. I also just moved my kettlebell & weights into my kitchen…. I will definitely use those daily now!

Dr. Phil Maffetone on the MAF Method

"I want to say one very, very important thing, which is that we're in this for fun. We're in this to be happy. There's nothing greater than being healthy and fit. With fitness, to see that we're now able to run at a faster pace at the same level of intensity, at the same heart rate, or generate more power, what a happy feeling that is being in a race and having fun. These are the things that bring happiness and are fun. We can't forget the fun part in all that we're doing."

Dr. Phil Maffetone is a pioneering figure in endurance sports and health science, implementing heart rate monitor training in the early '80s. As the originator of the MAF (Maximum Aerobic Function) Method and the 180 Formula, he has worked with elite athletes like six-time Hawaii Ironman World Champion Mark Allen. Having authored more than 20 books, including *The Big Book of Endurance Training and Racing*, Dr. Maffetone's holistic approach has influenced countless athletes worldwide, as he promotes the balance between health, happiness and athletic achievement.

Connect:
philmaffetone.com

Full Episodes:
extramilest.com/3
extramilest.com/8
extramilest.com/39
extramilest.com/68

The Formula for Health-First Training

Your training approach is centered on building an aerobic base first by using a heart rate monitor and running most of your runs at a relatively low heart rate. You developed the 180 Formula to calculate an athlete's maximum aerobic heart rate. What did you notice when athletes first started training this way?

The first thing I noticed was that the training many athletes were doing, including myself, coming from track and field, was not healthy. There were high injury rates, fatigue, and many athletes would drift into overtraining, which can lead to depression and a host of health problems. Training at higher heart rates was creating initially fit athletes who were unhealthy, and eventually, unhealthy athletes who were falling apart.

What I noticed early on was that the 220 formula wasn't a good way to evaluate or train because it resulted in a higher heart rate than necessary. I also noticed that athletes who were running with a lower heart rate had a better gait. They looked better when they were running.

The first significant finding was related to gait and biomechanics. When runners transitioned from a lower heart rate aerobic zone to a higher heart rate anaerobic zone, their biomechanics would deteriorate. This not only posed problems within a race but also throughout the season, leading to slower performance at the same heart rate, which is the opposite of what we want.

With the 180 Formula, I focused on the health of the athlete. Those who were healthier ended up with a higher heart rate, and those who were less healthy had lower heart rates. The 180 Formula provided a reliable way to establish a heart rate that would lead to a healthier, more efficient gait and improved overall health.

The problem with many runners, especially those who start later in life, is that they often skip essential steps in their development. It's like jumping from third grade to high school. It doesn't work because your brain and body don't develop efficiently.

Can you summarize the benefits of low heart rate training?

There are many benefits. One is that it builds the aerobic system. This involves the slow-twitch muscle fibers, which we're endowed with, much more than the fast-twitch anaerobic muscles.

The aerobic system is slow-twitch. They're muscle fibers that are associated with endurance. They not only allow us to run farther, but they allow us to sit at our desk without hurting our back. They support our joints and other muscles, ligaments, tendons, cartilage and everything else in a way that the anaerobic fast-twitch muscle fibers cannot do.

Some of your athletes have won races without doing any interval training or speed work. How important is anaerobic speed work?

We live in a no-pain, no-gain society where everyone thinks more is better. Speed is important, but it plays a minor role in endurance sports. In a marathon, 98% of your energy comes from the aerobic system. If that's the case, why spend so much time on anaerobic training, which plays a relatively minor role?

In the early '80s, I did a study with 223 runners who spent three to six months building their aerobic base with no weightlifting or anaerobic training. At the end of their base period, they ran a flat 5K, and 76% ran a personal best, despite being experienced runners. This suggests that aerobic training alone can lead to significant performance improvements.

Can you talk about that relationship between stress and aerobic running pace?

That's a very important issue. Stress affects us. It affects our brain, which then impairs fat burning. And so once we reduce the energy pipeline from fat, we can't perform as well. It's the opposite of what happens in the beginning when we start using MAF and we start eating better and training better, and we build up our fat burning.

In terms of stress, I always have to emphasize this because when we bring up that word "stress," it makes most people think of mental, emotional stress. But we also have physical stress, and we also have biochemical stress, which is where nutrition and metabolism come into play.

The bottom line is that stress impairs fat burning, which reduces our pace at the same heart rate. It reduces our power at the same heart rate. That overall also diminishes our health as well as fitness.

What would you say to someone experiencing challenges with low heart rate training, as many athletes have to slow down significantly at the beginning?

I just can't help saying to people, "If you're racing really well, if you're running some PRs, if your health is really good, if you're not injured, then keep doing what you're doing." But most people don't fall into that group. Most people have had injuries. They haven't had a PR in a long time. Decide that you're going to be healthy and fit, and then go about doing whatever you need to do to become healthier and more fit. It's really as simple as that.

I want you to learn how to individualize your health and individualize your training. I want you to learn how to best train. I want you to learn how much to eat for your particular needs. I've always been about self-health-management, self-care. How do I take care of myself?

Finding Your Flow

Some athletes get obsessed with heart rate training, cadence and stride length, which can bring added stress. Any thoughts for athletes who are unable to run relaxed or experience flow in their running?

What a great word you used: "flow." Flow is the ability to allow our brain to control things. We should be able to go out and run naturally, and running naturally means our brain knows what to do. We don't have to overthink it. We don't even have to think it. We just go out and run.

We're in a society where we're bombarded with all that information from the running magazines, from the website blogs, from our colleagues, from our training partners. But when we step out the door, it's time to turn all that off and flow, go with the flow, just run.

It's that simple. I often have to come back to the fact that humans get better naturally because their brain knows how to get better. Let your brain do it. Of course, you need a healthy brain, and it's particularly helpful when the body is healthy as well. And that fitness level will build automatically.

I heard you say that many athletes don't hit their aerobic peak until well into their forties. Can you talk more about this?

I think there's two ways to describe that. One is the generic approach with human physiology. You put it all together, and you seem to have a peak in the forties. And we see athletes who, as they get past what people think of as their prime—Mark Allen winning the Ironman—at a later age, are beating a lot of those young guys who were incredible athletes. Priscilla Welch won the New York City Marathon at age 42.

So the big question is, when did you begin this development? If you began at age 35 because you thought, "Okay, I gotta get off the couch and start training," and now you're running better and better, and at 45, you run a PR for your 10K or your marathon, well, there's a good chance you're going to run a PR at age 50 as well. It's conceivable you could run your best race and peak at age 55. I think the tradition of the peak is that we peak at age 25 or 30. That's a myth.

We Are What We Eat

One thing that stood out from your books is the dangers of processed carbs and refined sugars. What are some healthy alternatives?

Real food. People often don't know what real food is because we've been brainwashed by the media for so long. There are two types of food: junk food and healthy food. Junk food includes processed, packaged items like white flour, which is stripped of nutrients and filled with synthetic vitamins. Unfortunately, that's the foundation of many athletes' diets.

On the other hand, real food is unprocessed and nutrient-dense. Many people say they don't eat sugar, yet they consume packaged foods that contain hidden sugars. Being aware of real food and separating it from junk food is a crucial starting point.

The addiction part of junk food doesn't get talked about much. A lot of people would want to change and eat more healthily, yet it's so easy to just fall back into habits.

Yeah, well, the junk food companies long ago started to do something that was very important for their model: to make a lot of money, to sell a lot of junk food. Number one, they made junk food accessible, and so it was everywhere. So if you're going to help people get off junk food, you've got to resolve the issue of accessibility and cost.

"Addiction" technically may not be the correct word, but you can't tell someone who can't stop eating cookies or drinking Coke that they're not addicted. It's very painful. So we can call it technically anything we want, but it's really an addiction.

Rest and Recovery

Rest and sleep are crucial parts of training, yet many athletes don't get enough. Why is restful sleep so important, and how many hours do you recommend?

Healthy sleep usually means 7 to 9 hours of uninterrupted sleep. For someone running 50–60 miles (80–96 km) a week, 7 hours might not be enough. For a triathlete training 25 hours a week, closer to 9 hours might be necessary. Recovery is where we get most of our training benefits, not during the actual workout. If you're not recovering enough, you're building imbalances that will hinder your progress.

Stress hormones can wake people up in the middle of the night, which is a sign of serious problems. Eating right and balanced training can lower stress hormones and help you become a healthier, more fit athlete.

Can you explain the concept of the five-minute break?

The five-minute power break is a quick way to reduce stress and correct muscle imbalances. Injury rates are high in many sports, often due to muscle imbalances. If you can take five minutes to close your eyes and enter an alpha state, you can have a mini-therapy session for your brain and body. This reduces stress, balances blood sugar, improves fat burning and promotes overall health and fitness. You can do this anywhere, and it only takes five minutes.

Favorite Takeaways from Our YouTube Community

@CoachRobbBeams – Floris—I am new to your videos … absolutely love them. Dr. Maffetone literally saved my life; he talked me off the high-intensity, low-fat, low-sleep training cycles. Thanks to Dr. Maffetone, I have enjoyed 35-plus years of health, wellness and performance across all kinds of sports.

@shopkedai – "We can be fit and yet not healthy." I love the topic of recovery. My take is to never overstay in the Recovery Deficit Zone. We are in a way limited by how fast we can recover.

@standUpForTurtles – My favorite quote is "Humans get better naturally because our brains know how to get better." I love the idea that if I get out of the way and let my brain and body work together, they will optimize for a better solution.

@akashjalan4663 – I started MAF training 6 weeks ago and every day is a joy. … Life perspective has changed and there is more joy and happiness. … I have listened to every single podcast in your channel.

Lawrence van Lingen on Movement and Flow

"The purpose of running is to go where your heart calls you. Running should be a creative act of self-expression. If you can do that, you'll tend to make the right decisions, pick up on the right cues, and start following the right people."

Dr. Lawrence van Lingen is an extraordinarily influential movement specialist, originally from South Africa, who has been making waves in the endurance sports world. He's worked with some of the top athletes in the world to help them optimize their movement patterns and overall health. Lawrence's insights have completely transformed my own running and health, teaching me the power of fluidity and relaxation in both training and racing. *Triathlete* magazine featured an article titled, "Meet the Genius of Running Behind Jan Frodeno and Taylor Knibb's Comeback Stories. Why are already fast world champions flocking to Lawrence van Lingen to revamp their running form?" His unique approach, using tools like the flow rope and backward walking (see Chapter 11: Four Drills to Improve Your Running Form), unlocks new levels of running efficiency by focusing on proper hip extension and engagement of the posterior chain. He's all about mastering movement with mindfulness, and his work has had a profound impact on how athletes approach their performance and recovery.

Connect:
lawrencevanlingen.com

Full Episode:
extramilest.com/80

The Breakthrough: Transforming Running Through Awareness

After I started working with you a few years ago, through physical therapy, mobility and breathwork, I experienced a new level of relaxation and flow in my running. I sent you the following emotional video message: "Hey Lawrence, I just had a massive breakthrough of a run with the running technique you mentioned. The amount of relaxation into running right there, I've never experienced that before. Love you, brother." What happens with these types of breakthroughs athletes can experience?

Yes, I remember that video. That's what I live for. It's almost a spiritual journey. I don't know if you've got the whole stages of spiritual development. It's to basically become childlike again. That means you are the creator and author of your movement and your life.

Many people don't realize they're trapped, reflexive or stuck in patterns. Running happens on reflex. But again, is the tail wagging the dog, or is the dog wagging the tail? We talk about flow. I've had people that have swung the flow rope, and some people don't have an internal dialogue. I mean, I have an internal dialogue. It can drive me nuts sometimes, especially when trying to meditate. It just doesn't stop.

So they started swinging the rope, and they became aware of the internal dialogue. Or it got activated for the first time in their life, and they were 50. I've had people that became self-aware or started moving and said, "I never realized how hard I was on myself. I never realized how negative my internal dialogue was."

There is almost a sense of movement enlightenment or an awakening, for sure. People become self-aware in terms of movement, like it's a compartmentalized enlightenment or a compartmentalized awakening. You go, "Ooohhh," and then everything starts to shift. This can be so powerful.

With elite athletes now, I basically tell them that things might change and pre-warn them, especially if someone's at rock bottom. Generally speaking, people slowly improve. There's progress, not perfection. Things fall into place. It's normally not that dramatic, right? The way we work is pretty safe. In fact, there's an extraordinary element of not getting injured: how to do this safely; how to build you up, not break you down.

But let's say I work with a really good athlete, and they have a roadblock—an injury they can't overcome, and no one can help them. We know we need to change things around. I will literally warn them and say, "If you solve this problem and you start becoming more creative and reframe the way you're moving, how the world sees you will change, and how you see the world will change." That can be very disruptive. They'll ask, "What do you mean?" And it happens with coaches. Let's say we're working on extension, and you're suddenly thinking about pressing the ground away, the economy of movement, and relaxing into it. The less tension you have, the better you move.

I've helped people cure themselves of alcoholism, reconcile with their deceased mother—life-changing experiences. For me, running is far more than just running. Learning to run and move well is so rewarding. It's infinite, and it will engage you for the rest of your life. That's why children are so happy. They're obsessed with movement. Movement is meditation; it's what keeps them happy and engaged.

The Foundation: Rediscovering Natural Movement

Why do we know how to run so well as children, but then this changes over time? What are some of these changes people experience over the years, and what can people do to get back to that original fluid way of running?

Society imprints heavily on us, and we don't realize it. Like a fish in water, they don't know they're in water until you take them out. Culturally, there's a big narrative. In North America, it's a stiff spine culture. You must have backbone. You must stand for something. In Latin American countries, it's about salsa, belly dance or fluid movement. Culturally, just being in a certain environment shapes us more powerfully than we think.

Sitting is a huge factor. We're sitting longer, and from a young age. There's no doubt that screens massively impact this. When you stare at a screen, there's a thing called "screen apnea" or "email apnea." You hold your breath when you read an email because you're anticipating an event.

If you stare at a screen, your eyes fixate, and you're not looking far, wide, or using your eye movements. Eye movements are linked to the muscles at the back of your neck because that's how you track a bird or something that comes across your path. It's reflex. Just the fixation of your eyes will tighten up your back and hamstrings and shorten them. People get stuck out of the movement pattern from modern lifestyles.

Then there's physical, emotional and mental trauma. Some people fall on their tailbone and tighten up their pelvic floor and hip flexors, changing their gait pattern. Their knees come up, and they can literally have glute amnesia from falling on their butt.

We store negative emotions in flexion. Life can bear down on us, and we internalize things. There's that notion, then we spend so much time in flexion. The fetal position in the womb is a place of comfort, and it feels very natural for people. There's a huge psycho-emotional component to this. Kids are fearless, creative, expressive, with dreams and ambitions.

I did a thought exercise with someone recently. I said, "You used to be able to run, just remember." They were intrigued but didn't understand. I told them, "Sit down in a quiet space and go back to when you were happy and ran well because you know you ran really well. You had these dreams and ambitions." They said, "Oh my, I can remember running, the sensation of flying and being open." I said, "Go back, have a chat with that child, and check in on what your dreams and aspirations were like then." They said, "Oh my God, I was creative, inventive; I had all these ambitions." But life starts reacting to situations. You need to struggle; otherwise, you'll never grow. But a lot of people become reactive and reflexive, and their options shut down. They're not as creative as they used to be.

A fluid spine is a fluid mind: being creative, being the author of your movement, or moving proactively, choosing how you can move.

A lot of people are not the master of their movement. You can do this by doing a lot of reactive drills. What are you doing? You're reacting to an external stimulus in a very predictable pattern. We have reflex defensive pathways. Once our mind and body become reactive and defensive, our options narrow and shut down. There needs to be a state of play, a sense of creativity. People lose rhythm. Musically trained people will help them learn and rediscover running by learning to waltz or dance, putting rhythm into their running.

Humans are extraordinary. Who you surround yourself with, what the social media is showing—we see these elites doing fancy drills because they look good. We think we must imitate that, and that's how they got good. The reality is, they run a lot and run well. An elite athlete might do drills, and they don't get into their system as much because their overriding and dreaming ambition is to move forward, express themselves, and go forward in the world, which is drive.

But we, and I include myself, can sit there, react and copy because we are apes. We like to ape, get stuck and lose sight of what running is for. The purpose is to go where your heart calls you or to express or move forward through life.

A Strava study with 25,000 runners found that half of them either hate running or barely tolerate it, while only 8% love it. Unbelievable. Running is one of my greatest joys. My wish is to help people find and rediscover the joy as a healing experience.

The Practice: Relaxation and Breathing

One thing that has also helped me tremendously in my running is something you mentioned about pushing your feet into the ground. Instead of focusing so much on putting your foot in front, focus on pushing your feet into the ground. Can you talk through that more?

You should try to get your foot to land as close to under your hip as possible. You don't want your feet making ground contact in front of you. A huge part of that is getting your head on top of your shoulders and getting your arms back. If your head's forward, your feet will go forward. If your arms are forward, your feet will go forward. Posture will really help get your foot underneath your hip.

Super Shoes are designed so you're going to compress the shoe and spring out of them like a pogo stick. I think it's really helping a lot of people's running form, including elites, because people are starting to experience energy return and efficiency or elasticity in their running. We got into a muscle phase where you muscle through running and work your engine, your cardiovascular system, and there's a big focus on muscling it. One of the reasons why I think people should cue on pressing the earth backward is that it's a very powerful cue of moving from the center out.

Also, if you want to run fast in Super Shoes, you need to compress them into the ground and use the elastic spring to aid your running. Moving from the center out is also why we press the earth away. Then, it's hip drive. Many people try to improve their running mechanics by working on cadence. Most people increase their cadence by picking their feet up off the ground. I personally don't work on cadence—hardly ever—because cadence is a central movement pattern problem. I'd rather you swing the flow rope, learn to move from the hips, learn to generate power from where it's supposed to. The cadence will come.

In all movement lessons in the world, we understand you practice slowly, and the speed and power come. Most of the work we do is slow walking or slowing things down. That's the quickest way to teach your nervous system how to do things. If you do things quickly, you'll do them the same way you always did them. You'll go back to your reflex paths. There's a huge component of learning things slowly and letting the speed and power come.

The Mental Game: Presence and Racing

You've mentioned that sometimes when we do speed work, run at higher intensity, or race, it's the anticipation of what's to come that makes it challenging. You and I have spoken several times about being present; being here now. Often as athletes, we are disconnected from the present moment.

Yeah, that'll get into the perception of time, which I love. Let's talk about the psycho-emotional. You can't separate motion from emotion. How you move is how you feel. That's why it matters so much—the cues you choose, how you perceive running—because it impacts how you feel. And how we feel is all we ever worry about.

If I say, "Oh my, there's my ultimate joy underneath the Christmas tree. I'm so excited, and I want to get to it." I run over there, anticipating, thinking, "What's in the box? I want what's in the box." I'm getting ahead of myself. We now place so much significance on an event that we perceive will change our life. We think we can have all these good things if we do that thing. But the reality is, we only have the here and now. You open that box, and it might be the wrong toy, and then it's not so amazing.

The step you're making now, if you make that as well as you can, will set you up for success in the future. That very powerful reframing, if you get it right, is one of the most powerful endurance cues you can use. I've seen people have really good races simply because of how they're framing their mental and emotional state, and their ability to stay in the moment is very powerful.

We'll take this back to our perception of time. When you swing the rope, and you've taught people how to swing the rope, many people rush, can't slow down, can't stop and can't listen. I'll make them aware of this moment and say, "Can you see that you're rushing and going on to the next thing?" When you start swinging the rope backward and create movement options, you start reframing things, creating a sense of more time and space. It's one reason I don't like working on cadence. It makes you feel you don't have enough time. You're not taking enough steps per minute. You should take more steps per minute. It makes you feel rushed, anxious. In the military, they say, "Slow is smooth, smooth is fast," or in triathlon transitions, "Don't make mistakes."

Many people working on cadence try to take enough steps per minute. As soon as your foot hits the ground, you have to pick it back up. You don't have a sense of rolling your foot, relaxing forward, flourishing off your toes, hip drive, because time is narrow for you. That lack of time in your sympathetic nervous system creates a sense of anxiety. Your breathing rate will be higher than it should be. Your blood lactate won't be what it could be. You might find your digestion doesn't work as well as it could. All of these things start to link and sync up together. When you get it right, it's luminal, transcendent; it can be incredibly powerful.

The literature and science are obsessed with rigidity, bracing, guarding. But again, that puts you in a reactive state. You're not the author of your movement. We need these things. You need to be able to react, to brace or stiffen. But you can't live in a guarded, braced, stiffened state. Your movement becomes segmented, choppy. You're not getting the best out of your muscles. If your shoulders are up near your ears, when your diaphragm and pelvic floor are tight, you have to relax your diaphragm and pelvic floor. When you learn to rotate your shoulders, they should swap from side to side because your hips are animated. If your hips are empowered and animated, your shoulders will swap when you're running.

Another thing, common knowledge is to keep your hips still when you run. No, they should be animated and have contralateral movement. They do this weird figure-of-eight dance, which is extraordinary. I still haven't figured it out. What happens is your shoulders will animate, and you'll see that in really good runners.

There are so many people doing skips, shortening the hamstrings and contracting the hamstrings, or there's a narrative of "my hamstrings are biceps, and you should contract them." I like to think of hamstrings as "ham-springs." If you're driving with length, you'll actually stretch the hamstring. It's contracting as well. It's doing two things at once. You'll see in elite athletes that run really well, their back leg goes dead straight.

In challenging moments in a race, it's so important we still find ways to relax. Share your thoughts on relaxation while running.

Yeah, and get back into the moment. I mean, we were having this conversation with Taylor Knibb. I explained this in preparation for Kona. I call it the "Oh my word" moment in a marathon. The "Oh my word" part of an Ironman marathon is when you go, "Oh my word, this is a lot." It's almost like you wake up.

You're swimming, biking, running, doing all the things, and it's all going fine. Then at some pivotal moment, you go, "Oh my word, I've got 12 Ks to go," or whatever it is. That's a lot. And right now, I'm having a lot of sensations. Generally speaking, that's when you start thinking about how far you've gone, what your pace was, what you've been doing. You start thinking, "How far do I have to go?" You're pulled out of being in the moment.

The anticipation of what's to come leads many people to hit the wall, not just a nutrition or training thing. Immediately, you should get present, get in the moment. Don't think about how far you've gone. Think about how well you're doing, and do what you can in the moment to set yourself up for the next step. That can often take the tension out of it.

Mantras at this stage are very important. Your internal dialogue: You'll notice bad movement and bad internal dialogue go together. So immediately work on a positive mental dialogue and reframing. You should talk to yourself in the second person at this stage. You should be saying, "Flo, you're awesome. Flo, you're in the moment."

Know your "why" before you're doing ultra-endurance or Ironman. Don't, in that moment, suddenly think, "Oh, I need to think of a reason to get to the finish line." You need to have that preloaded. That's why many people run for charities or causes greater than themselves. Humans have that in them. If you're doing well, I mean, you can do it for any distance race, but particularly for ultra-distance races or longer races, or the marathon.

Know why, when it gets tough, you're going to push through. I don't think you need to be tougher than other people. There's a lovely Boston study showing that the tougher you think you are, the more of a pain game you think a marathon is, and the more prepared you are to suffer. That's the best predictor of slowing down in the second half and ending up suffering more. I'm not saying don't be tough or hard. I'm saying have your "why." Know why, when it gets tough, you're going to carry on running, and have that figured out before. Because when you're in the middle of a race, that's not the time to start figuring out your "why."

Any closing thoughts or advice for runners looking to become stronger, healthier and happier athletes?

Running should be a creative act of self-expression. If you can do that, you'll tend to make the right decisions, pick up on the right cues and start following the right people. The world, the universe, is like social media. If I create a blank account and seek out hate, violence and strong opinions, trying to reinforce my belief system on social media, the world will just project that straight back at me. We need to shape our reality, be the creators and authors of our movement and take back control. It requires bravery and courage.

Remember, be patient with yourself. Running is a journey, and the more you understand your body, the better you'll feel in your running.

Many people have been hurt or traumatized, don't want to feel, are shutting off or are overwhelmed and can't feel. It's a courageous act of creativity that you need to undertake. Start thinking along those lines. I strongly suggest you read Rick Rubin's book *The Creative Act* because he seems to have distilled these really complex concepts and made them actionable.

Rubin has a beautiful gift of describing how reality works. Live your life as an artist and create. That means courage. You're the authority of movement.

You create your movement. Learn to trust your body in your movement. You might need a guiding framework on that journey, which is what I'm trying to provide. But that's the way, and that's how we will change the world for the better, one person and one runner at a time.

Favorite Takeaways from Our YouTube Community

@gwenne2377 – This. BLEW. My. Mind. I'm almost giving up on running and dreading training because I signed up for a triathlon this year. Everything discussed here resonates—emotion and motion, the nervous system, inner dialogue, and the peak lesson for me is authentic self-expression. I believe we're all here to remember our authentic selves and express it—that is the highest state of being!

@lucycartwright9053 – "The purpose of running is to go where your heart calls you." I loved hearing this. It really speaks to why I run and reminded me of a peak experience I had running in the hills of north Wales, years ago, where I felt as light as air and that the mountains were a giant playground which I was free to explore.

@CLARE238 – This has to be one of your best interviews, Floris ... what a find ... you and Lawrence have helped me fall in love with running again ... I'd given up on myself ... following menopause ... Covid ... long Covid ... I've got fresh Hope. Thank you. 🙏

@Anza_34832 – Thanks for bringing up Lawrence van Lingen and his flow rope exercises! I watched your video five months ago and practiced it ever since: My running movement has improved, swinging my hips, running with less effort, not having a stiff lower back afterwards and recovering faster.

@MelanieSakowski – "To be childlike again; to be the creator and author of your life." I feel like the silence after finishing a really good book's last sentence, closing it and looking around hoping to share that awe.

Patrick McKeown on Breathwork

"Many children and adults persistently mouth breathe; they breathe fast, they breathe upper chest, and they have their mouths open during sleep. From a biochemistry point of view, they don't have optimal breathing. This results in their blood vessels constricting and less oxygen delivery."

Patrick McKeown, author of *The Oxygen Advantage*, is an expert in breathing techniques. His teachings show how proper breathing enhances athletic performance and health. Discovering methods to manage his asthma and improve sleep, Patrick emphasizes optimal breathing to boost oxygen uptake, sleep quality and athletic performance.

Connect:
oxygenadvantage.com

Full Episode:
extramilest.com/30

Breathing Fundamentals

What's the correct way to breathe?

Many people develop bad habits, and there's a lot of misinformation about breathing. When considering breathing, we need to think about how to improve oxygen uptake in the blood and oxygen delivery to the cells, to open up the airways and influence the automatic functioning of the body. Many children and adults persistently breathe through their mouths, breathe quickly and use their upper chest. They sleep with their mouths open, leading to poor oxygen delivery, constricted blood vessels and poor functional movement, increasing the risk of injury. When we talk about breathing, we must consider its impact on emotions, sleep and physical exercise. And remember, less is often more when it comes to breathing.

When I first tried nasal breathing during runs, my nose got runny, and I felt dizzy. Why does this happen?

When you first switch to nasal breathing during exercise, it's tough because you're going from breathing through a larger space (your mouth) to a smaller one (your nose). The nose imposes resistance, which is actually beneficial because it slows down your breathing. Mouth breathing leads to greater water loss, upper chest activation, reduced oxygen uptake and trauma to the airways. During nasal breathing, carbon dioxide levels in the blood increase, leading to greater air hunger. This sensation is a sign that your body is adapting to the higher levels of carbon dioxide, which ultimately improves oxygen delivery to your muscles.

What's a nasal dilator, and how does it help?

A nasal dilator is a small device that helps open up the nasal passages. If you press your fingers on either side of your nostrils and gently pull them apart, you'll find it easier to breathe. A nasal dilator works similarly by physically expanding the nostrils, making it easier to breathe through your nose, especially during exercise. Some people, like me, have structural issues that make nasal breathing more challenging, so a nasal dilator can be quite helpful.

George Dallam studied athletes who nasal-breathed for six months. What were his findings?

George Dallam is a triathlete and academic who conducted a study on nasal breathing. After six months, the athletes' respiratory rate during nasal breathing was 39 breaths per minute, compared to 49 breaths per minute with mouth breathing. They also had a 22% reduction in ventilation while maintaining the same work rate intensity. This means they achieved the same performance with 22% less breathlessness. This study highlights the efficiency and benefits of nasal breathing during exercise.

Adapting to Nasal Breathing

What's your view on mouth taping during sleep?

Mouth taping is about ensuring you don't breathe through your mouth during sleep. When you sleep with your mouth open, your tongue is more likely to fall back into the airway, narrowing it and increasing the resistance to breathing. This can lead to snoring, sleep apnea and other sleep-related issues. Mouth taping helps maintain nasal breathing, which improves sleep quality and reduces stress on the heart. If you're waking up with a dry mouth, it's a sign that you're mouth breathing during sleep, which can lead to poor sleep quality and feeling tired in the morning.

How important is nasal breathing during sleep?

Nasal breathing during sleep is crucial for maintaining good health. Dr. Christian Guilleminault, who coined the term "obstructive sleep apnea," was a strong advocate for nasal breathing during sleep. For children, persistent mouth breathing can negatively affect their academic ability, cognitive development, facial structure and airway development. For adults, nasal breathing during sleep ensures a more restful sleep, reduces the risk of sleep apnea and helps you wake up feeling more refreshed.

How should advanced athletes incorporate nasal breathing in training?

Nasal breathing should be incorporated gradually, especially for advanced athletes. I would recommend doing about 50% of your training with your mouth closed to build up respiratory strength and improve overall breathing efficiency. The other 50% can be done with mouth breathing to maintain intensity. Nasal breathing during warm-ups can also help increase oxygen delivery to the muscles and calm the mind, preparing you for the workout ahead. It's about finding a balance and gradually increasing your capacity to breathe through your nose at higher intensities.

Favorite Takeaways from Our YouTube Community

@chloeanddiego – My biggest takeaway from this is just how much of our "success" as athletes is connected to what we do in everyday life when we are not training. Traditionally, I would have correlated my success only to what I could do in the gym and not thought to make significant changes to what my body is doing during the majority of my day.

@joanslominski4220 – "Nose breathing at night can increase deep sleep" was my big takeaway.

@stephendurley1239 – I liked that he said we could breathe 20% less with the same effort after we get fully adapted. I've been a mouth breather for my adult life and have had to really work hard to focus to nose breathe all day. After 3 months I've had significant improvements in my sleep quality and have worked up to several miles a week nasal breathing while running. The journey continues! Thank you, Floris, for bringing this subject to endurance athletes! Your podcasts have had a huge impact on my life; can't thank you enough!

@affordableplumbingandelect2119 – I used to suffer chronic sleep apnea, but then I heard someone talking about nose breathing on the radio, and actually taping your mouth at night. What a life saver this was for me. It literally stopped my snoring, improved my sleep time 100% and saved my marriage.

Kasper van der Meulen on Conscious Breathing

"For athletes, especially runners, the most important thing, I think, is to use breath to gain a deeper body awareness and a higher ability to gauge where you are at in relation to your maximum and minimum."

Kasper van der Meulen is an expert in human performance, breathwork and mindfulness. Through barefoot ultramarathons, cold exposure and continuous experimentation, he combines ancient practices with modern science to help athletes reach their full potential.

Connect:
instagram.com/kaspersfocus

Full Episode:
extramilest.com/74

The Benefits of Breathwork

What are some benefits of practicing breathwork regularly?

What I love about breathwork is that it offers compound benefits, meaning ever-increasing benefits without necessarily increasing effort. A common thread among my students is the increased ability to regulate their state. For example, if your head is racing at night, you can take three conscious breaths and check, "Oh yeah, I actually feel calmer now."

Breathing is something you can do on autopilot your entire life and never consciously explore. But considering athletes breathe heavily for hours weekly, it's worth asking, "What if tweaking breath slightly creates performance improvements?"

A Simple Technique for Runners

If you could recommend something tangible runners could easily implement, what would it be?

I think the highest leverage thing for any athlete is improving CO_2 tolerance. The most effective way to do this is hypoventilation, or under-breathing. Simply tune in to your breathing and reduce it to "not quite enough," creating a feeling called "air hunger." For two minutes, relax your muscles and calm your mind despite the discomfort, then return to normal breathing.

This increases CO_2 and reduces available oxygen, improving cellular oxygen use. Endurance athletes can do the same work with fewer breaths or more work with the same amount of breathing.

Beginners should first enjoy running and build mileage. But advanced athletes can benefit greatly, as this adds valuable training without extra physical stress, helping prevent overtraining and injury.

Staying Calm in Tough Moments

At the later stages of a marathon, runners often struggle with breathing. Any advice for keeping control during those tough moments?

It's inevitable to hit tough moments in marathons, but timing matters. In the end, controlling your exhale is crucial. Two equally exhausted runners differ greatly if one controls their exhale while the other gasps erratically. Controlled exhaling gives an edge.

A great tip is to sync your breathing with your steps. For example, two steps in, two steps out, focusing on your exhale. If you can keep this rhythm, you'll enter a trancelike state, where all your focus is on coordinating breath and movement. This also enhances the runner's high, keeping your mind off the discomfort.

Finding a strategy that works for you, instead of letting your breath do whatever, can help you maintain control in those final miles. It's not foolproof, but it's one way to stay in control.

Any closing thoughts for athletes aiming to become stronger, healthier and happier?

Focus on having fun and training in a way that brings you joy, peace and meaning in the moment. Life is short. You could be chasing your ultimate marathon time and still get hit by a bus. Instead of constantly thinking about future goals, enjoy the process now. Many athletes think, "I need to be better," but remember, you have this amazing biological machine that can experience incredible things. So why not enjoy it? Don't take performance too seriously. Treat your body well, and the performance will naturally follow.

Favorite Takeaways from Our YouTube Community

@liamfinnegan8085 – Out of breath is out of control of breath. That's a great quote.

@Rls2236 – Love the part about how breathwork can help improve fitness and function without additional impact or damage to the body.

@alangray8952 – Great conversation; liked the advice about aligning breath to steps. Going to try that out; think it will be a good way of staying under control.

@dsfrye01 – I really appreciate the thought of horizontal breathing. Utilizing the diaphragm is so important, and this is a wonderful cue.

Jennifer Schmidt on Mental Health

"You want to improve as an athlete, you can't think of your mental health as being this isolated thing that isn't going to improve your performance. When you start addressing all of the underlying issues in your body, your sport performance is going to go up substantially. If you fix it from the root, you are actually going to see improvements in your sport and your times, and your pace is just going to come without technically any extra physical effort."

Jennifer Schmidt is an athlete mental-health coach who believes addressing mental health is key to unlocking athletic performance. Through her own journey, Jennifer discovered that mental health deeply connects to physical well-being, especially gut health. Her holistic approach helps athletes manage emotional highs and lows, encouraging kindness to oneself and awareness of mental health's impact on performance.

Connect:
igniteyourhealth.ca

Full Episode:
extramilest.com/73

Balancing Mental and Physical Health

What are some common challenges athletes face around mental health?

The recognition piece is key. Many athletes, especially in endurance sports, just keep increasing their training, whether it's doing longer races or trying to get faster and stronger. It's a coping mechanism. While exercise does have mental health benefits, there's a point where pushing the boundaries becomes a red flag. I start asking questions when I see athletes constantly increasing their training load. It's important to understand why you're doing it.

Look at your life and see what's happening at the times when you're having these thoughts. How are you feeling before and after training sessions? Are you still getting that runner's high, or are you just chasing it, thinking that doing more will get you there? Athletes should pay attention to these signals when considering whether there's a mental health issue at play.

Overcoming Stress and Anxiety

What practical methods can athletes use to manage anxiety?

There are two sides to anxiety management. One is in-the-moment management. Whether you struggle with ongoing anxiety or just have moments of it, you need to learn how to manage it as it happens. Managing it involves cueing your body that it's safe. Anxiety is basically your body perceiving a threat. You want to stimulate the vagus nerve, which touches most of the organs in your body, to shift from a fight-or-flight state to a rest-and-digest state.

Deep breathing, gentle exercise (like walking), yoga, stretching, getting outside in nature, all these cue your body that it's safe. Gratitude is another powerful tool; it's the antidote to anxiety. It expands your vision beyond the immediate threat. Managing anxiety in the moment is essential, but if you struggle with it regularly, you need to address the underlying issues. Gut health, nervous system regulation, inflammation all play a role.

You Are More than a Runner

How can athletes deal with injuries without getting depressed or losing their identity?

The identity piece is crucial. As much as sport is part of who we are, it's important not to tie your whole identity to it. When you're injured, you might not be able to do any sport. So, I challenge athletes to expand their recreation interests beyond sport. Explore creative activities like art, music or writing. Even if you're not good at it, having other interests gives you something to do when you're injured. This way, you're not solely relying on sport for your sense of self and well-being.

What are your thoughts on journaling as part of an athlete's training journey, not just for injured athletes?

Journaling is powerful. There are many styles, but one of the most effective for athletes is stream-of-consciousness writing. This method helps you get past your conscious thoughts and tap into your subconscious, allowing you to problem solve from a deeper place. It's more than just venting. It's about challenging yourself and gaining new perspectives. Gratitude journaling is another effective practice. Gratitude is the antidote to anxiety, but it needs to be practiced regularly, just like training.

What advice do you have for athletes who feel down or lost after a race?

The post-race blues are common because, during training, you're getting dopamine hits from achieving your goals. When the race is over, those dopamine hits stop, and you can feel lost. To combat this, find other sources of dopamine: Get outside; connect with nature and set new goals, even if they're not sport-related. It's about finding balance and keeping yourself motivated.

Favorite Takeaways from Our YouTube Community

@Hillrunner50 – I appreciate that she brought up numerous factors to consider when thinking about mental health, one of them being gut health. Many people don't realize how much what they put into their bodies on a daily basis makes a huge impact on their well-being.

@krisa.1263 – My favorite takeaway is to manage anxiety in the moment by stimulating the vagus nerve—deep breathing, walking, stretching & gratitude.

@robthompson4882 – Reflecting on the value of developing a nonathletic hobby/pursuit to be able to manage mental health at time of a physical injury/setback and so having an activity to complement my running that is not athletically based.

@jenniferkellett4314 – "Experience the present!" On my Friday-evening run three pelicans flew overhead towards the sunset, and I just stopped in awe at the beauty—no grappling for my phone—just enjoyed the special moment.

Susan Piver on Meditation

"The basic technique could not be more simple. It's you, sitting on this earth, breathing. But the objective is to notice how and who you are right now, from moment to moment."

Susan Piver is a meditation expert, teacher and *New York Times* bestselling author. She founded the Open Heart Project, the world's largest virtual mindfulness community. Susan has taught thousands worldwide and has authored nine books, including *Start Here Now: An Open-Hearted Guide to the Path and Practice of Meditation*.

Connect:
susanpiver.com

Full Episode:
extramilest.com/6

Understanding Meditation Basics

What is meditation really, and how can runners benefit from it?

It's actually very simple. Meditation asks you to take your primary attention off your thoughts and place it on another object instead. In most common practices, including the one I teach, that object is your breath. It's very convenient, you're already doing it anyway, it's always right where you are, and you don't have to introduce anything new.

Your attention will stray back into thought because you can't stop thinking. When your attention strays, you notice that, and that's a wonderful moment of wakefulness. You gently let go and bring your attention back to the breath. That's it.

The objective is to notice how and who you are right now, moment to moment. That's called relaxing. Normally, we push ourselves to accomplish more or sometimes to slow down. But we're still pushing. The practice says, "Stop pushing and just be with yourself as you are."

How long would a normal practice be for someone starting out with meditation? Would five or ten minutes a day consistently for five days a week be a good start?

Beyond a good start, it would be a fabulous start! Five to ten minutes a day, Monday to Friday, is great. It's better than doing an hour every once in a while. The important thing with meditation, as with any habit, is consistency. If you run a mile every day for five days, you will get somewhere. But if you try to run 5 miles (8 km) in one day, you could hurt yourself.

What are some of the benefits you experience from meditation?

One of the primary benefits is that you notice what your mind is on and what your body is doing, whether it's running or riding a bike. Suddenly, you notice that your mind and body are synchronized, and that's what mindfulness is: when mind and body are in the same place, and you're actually attending to what you're doing without being elsewhere.

Meditation is a spiritual practice. It is not just a self-help technique, even though neuroscience confirms many benefits: lower stress hormones, better immunity, improved sleep and chronic pain management. These benefits have been recognized for over 2,500 years.

The real benefits are what Buddhist thought calls the three qualities of the awakened mind: compassion, wisdom and power, meaning presence. A surge of power comes with that—not aggression, but strength, endurance, resilience, curiosity and creativity. Interestingly, these benefits arise most quickly when you abandon your agenda entirely and look for the real, unconditioned experiences.

What obstacles do people encounter when starting meditation?

The primary obstacle is mismanaged expectations for one's practice. Like, "I'm going to sit down, put on my yoga pants, look really happy, and all my problems will melt away." Actually, meditation broadens your emotional spectrum, so you feel more, not less.

The classic obstacle in Buddhism is called laziness, and there are three kinds. First is ordinary laziness: "I'll just watch TV instead." Second is becoming disheartened: losing confidence in yourself and the practice. Third is being "too busy," which means if you're too busy for what's truly important. If you're too busy to maintain your health, relationships and creativity, then you've become lazy about your priorities.

Meditation for Runners

How does meditation specifically help with endurance sports?

Whether physical or emotional, the ability to remain with your experience is crucial. When we fight discomfort by thinking about something else, it only comes back stronger. Instead, there's a way of relaxing with what's uncomfortable. You can acknowledge your pain: "Okay, you're here too, knee pain, lungs, muscles, here we go; we're doing this together."

My teacher completed the Boston Marathon and shared how at mile 20 (32 km), he began working with his mind using meditation techniques. By visualizing what was happening in his joints and applying his meditation practice, he finished successfully despite the pain.

I've noticed while running the Boston Marathon that my facial expressions became grumpy. Once I told myself to relax and smile, I got a boost of energy. It's really about being more aware of your body.

Exactly. Being able to work with your attention. You described that so well. You first noticed the grumpy face or whatever it was, and that's the key: to notice it. Otherwise, it just reads in your inner experience as some kind of discomfort. But when you can pinpoint it, "Oh, it's my face, or my shoulders," then you have a choice. You don't have any choice without awareness; whatever is riding you, you're not riding it. But once you've taken it in with your awareness, your options open up. You can think, "What would it be like to have relaxed shoulders? What would it feel like to have a relaxed face?" Then you can let go and shift your attention from your body to the people around you or what's going on behind you. That ability to direct your attention where you want it to go is mindfulness.

Do you have recommendations for becoming more mindful while running?

Make your body running the object of your meditation. Place your attention on what it feels like when your feet hit the ground, when the air is on your skin—just some aspect of what you're doing.

When you take running itself as your meditation, it creates a more interesting, sustained connection to your practice. If you constantly distract yourself with music or other things, that can become stressful. But if you make your running experience your meditation, it becomes joyful, with both physical and spiritual benefits.

Favorite Takeaways from Our YouTube Community

@RameshPatel-kd4iq – Make running part of meditation and experience your true essence.

@ajaykhajuria1927 – The takeaway for me in this video is there are three types of laziness: ordinary laziness, disheartened laziness and too busy laziness.

@oga-h7480 – I do agree with how meditation helps your running performance. Meditating is such a healthy resource.

Scott Warr and Don Freeman on Trail Running

*"Our pace changes, but our workload is even.
That's the art of trail running."*

Scott Warr and Don Freeman host *Trail Runner Nation*, the world's #1 trail-running podcast. Their humor, passion for the sport and easygoing style make every episode feel like a conversation with friends. Through stories, practical tips and insights from top athletes and experts, they inspire runners to push their limits while enjoying the journey. It was their podcast in 2013 where I first heard about low heart rate training, which changed my life.

Connect:
trailrunnernation.com

Full Episode:
extramilest.com/61

The Art of Trail Running

What were those first trail runs like for you guys when you first started out and transitioned from road running to trail running?

Don Freeman: When I first started on the trail, I was full of questions. Do you run this hill? How much? I was running with Dana Gard, one of my mentors. I noticed that I was running behind Dana, and I thought this guy doesn't know what he's doing. Downhill, we're bombing; through the flats, just shuffling along; through the ups, hard hiking.

Then I learned, as the day went on, he knows exactly what he's doing. Our pace changes, but our workload is even. That's when it dawned on me: That's the art of trail running. It's keeping your workload even no matter what trail you're on. Up, down, flat, your workload's even.

Getting Started on Trails

What small steps can someone take to experience trail running for the first time?

Scott Warr: There are so many apps now to find trails regardless of where you are. GPS watches bring safety. You're less worried if you fall or get hurt. Go to your local running store and just ask them. They know where the clubs are. There may be a Tuesday evening running club that goes out to the trails, and I think that's a good way to start.

Don Freeman: The running community is supportive. If you show up at that store or the trailhead for one of those trail runs, they're going to put their arms around you and make you feel welcome.

The Mental Game

Our minds are very powerful tools. How do you view the mental component of running?

Don Freeman: I love talking about the mental side of running. It's the whole sport. It's wrapped up in just that nugget, that moment, that internal discussion you have with yourself. "Oh, this is hard. No, I can do it. I need to change this so I can make it happen." There are so many things around the mental game, the ball that bounces around inside your cranium.

That piece fascinates me. It can take you out of a race; it can put you into a race. You'll get to learn who you really are. You'll get to meet the "you" inside of you. The mental game is like flying an airplane. You have all these dials out in front of you, and you kind of have to monitor each one of those dials.

Advancing to Ultras

Do you have any recommendations for anyone wanting to get into the ultrarunning distance?

Don Freeman: Just keep the workload easy. It should never be hard. If it's hard, back off because you can't do something hard for a long time. Find where you feel comfortable, stay in that zone, and then watch the magic happen. The body is very good at doing things for a long time if you set it up right, as long as you don't sabotage yourself. You can sabotage yourself with pace, electrolytes, hydration, not having the right footwear, getting a blister, no chafing prevention. There are a lot of ways to sabotage yourself. Don't sabotage yourself. Make it easy; go long.

Balance and Self-Care

Many listeners are recreational runners with regular jobs, looking to improve as athletes. Any final advice for becoming stronger, healthier and happier?

Scott Warr: Sometimes I have to be on a work call in the early mornings, and I can't get out and do my morning run. What I did that really helps me is a week before, I go and block off times for runs on my work calendar, so other people can't sabotage that time. That's been a real help for me.

Don Freeman: I think people should be compassionate with themselves. Don't be so hard on yourself. There are peaks and valleys in life, and one of the things we've learned from talking to people is there's such a thing as emotional stress, and that weighs on you. You can't always measure how well you're doing by looking at a watch. Sometimes you just need to go out there and enjoy it. Be compassionate with yourself. Let it be an easy run, a slow run. Don't judge yourself, just enjoy yourself. I think that's probably one of the most important takeaways I've learned.

Scott Warr: Most of us are Type A personalities, and if we miss a run, we beat ourselves up about it. Again, a lesson I learned from David Roche is, I would say, "Hey, I didn't get out there, but I'm going to take that and move it to tomorrow, which is my rest day." He goes, "Nope, no, you're not. That's in the past. Forget about it. Tomorrow is your rest day. Rest, then get back on your schedule." That grace, if you miss something because of whatever, give yourself some grace.

Favorite Takeaways from Our YouTube Community

@coolingrid – I love TRN. Discipline trumps motivation anytime.

@beerandchips2545 – "Be compassionate with yourself." I really needed to hear that today. I listened to the podcast while I was skiing, and I had to take a break for a moment when your guest said that line. Cheers.

@chadhawkinsart – I love the advice to block off workout time on your work calendar. That's a great idea!

@inyofasa29 – Your actions reinforce your identity, and your identity reinforces your actions. Decide the kind of person you want to be—a runner, a good dad, a hard worker—and start the virtuous cycle.

Andy Blow on Hydration and Fasting

"The best endurance athletes aren't just the fittest. They're the ones who dial in their hydration and fueling strategy. You can be as fit as you like, but if you get your fluid, sodium or carb intake wrong, your performance will suffer. When you get these elements right, you give yourself the best chance to perform at your peak."

Andy Blow is the founder of Precision Fuel & Hydration, and a leading expert in sports hydration and fueling strategies. A former elite triathlete and sports scientist, Andy has worked with top endurance athletes to optimize hydration, sodium intake and race day nutrition. His insights have helped thousands of runners, triathletes and cyclists avoid cramping, fatigue and performance crashes.

Connect with Andy:
precisionhydration.com

Episode:
extramilest.com/64

Getting Hydration and Fueling Right

What are common fueling mistakes athletes make, and how can runners avoid them?

There are a lot of mistakes when it comes to long races and fueling. The most common mistake is not knowing how much energy you need to consume. A lot of people go into a race with a vague idea. Maybe they'll eat when they feel hungry or eat a bit more or less than last time, but they don't have a solid grasp on the numbers required for different race distances and times.

The key distinction is between calories and carbohydrates. We talk almost exclusively about grams of carbs per hour because that's the fuel your body burns at high intensity. One gram of fat has 9 calories; 1 gram of protein or carbohydrate has 4, but you're relying on carbs for endurance. You could eat a block of butter for calories, but it won't help your performance.

For efforts under two hours, most people need 30 to 60 grams of carbs per hour, just enough to keep blood sugar stable and avoid brain fade, since you've got a lot of stored glycogen in your muscles. But once you go beyond that two-hour mark, especially past three hours, you start burning through glycogen, and your performance drops. That's when we look at 60 grams per hour, sometimes 90 grams, and for elite athletes in long, high-intensity races, even up to 120 grams per hour. Most people will fall somewhere in the middle, with the number increasing the longer and harder the effort.

Many runners assume they're fueling enough in training and racing, but when we have closely analyzed the intake of some of the runners in our Personal Best Program, several of them are not taking in enough. At the Chicago Marathon I took in 90 grams of carbs per hour. There is a fine line between fueling enough and risking stomach issues. Can you talk about that balance?

Yes, great point. In the '80s and '90s, marathoners often ran on nothing, believing they should train to resist fuel intake. The concern was that taking in too much would cause GI distress. But over time, research and experience have shown that the more carbs you can absorb and metabolize, the more energy you'll have to sustain a faster pace.

Like anything in training, fueling needs practice. You can't expect to suddenly take in three gels per hour on race day and feel fine; it's like expecting to run 20 miles (32 km) at goal pace without buildup. The digestive system gets compromised at higher intensities since blood is redirected to working muscles. That's why it's crucial to train your gut in the weeks leading up to a race.

How should athletes train their gut for fueling? Should they practice during long runs or at higher intensity?

The best time to train it is in your longest, hardest runs. That does three things: It helps your gut tolerate more fuel, supports performance by driving better adaptation and speeds up recovery by preventing deep glycogen depletion. For marathoners, these key runs usually happen every two or three weeks, and that's when you should really push your carb intake.

If you're not used to consuming a lot of carbs, start incorporating gels or sports drinks into medium-to-long runs once or twice a week, especially in the last eight to ten weeks before race day. The key is starting early, even when you don't feel like it. You also need to get comfortable carrying, opening and consuming fuel while running hard.

Hot conditions make it harder to absorb calories because blood is redirected to the skin for cooling. In cold races, athletes sometimes under-fuel because they can't open their gels or don't feel thirsty.

Let's talk about fueling choices. In ultraraces, athletes often take in solid foods during walk breaks, but in a marathon or half-marathon, you want something easily digestible. How have energy gels evolved, and what makes them effective for quick absorption?

That's a great point. In longer, lower-intensity events, solid foods can work because you're missing meals and need something to settle your stomach. Food is also a big morale booster in ultras. But in shorter endurance events like marathons, liquid carbohydrates are your best bet because they're easy to consume while running hard. If formulated well, they pass through the stomach quickly into the bloodstream.

Gels sit between these extremes. Elites often rely on personal bottles, but for most marathon runners, gels are a convenient, concentrated fuel source. Some can be taken without water, while others need to be washed down. Sports drinks, gels and chews are designed for rapid absorption. They're pure fuel with no fiber, fat or protein to slow digestion.

Our products, for example, use a blend of glucose and fructose. This is key when pushing intake beyond 60 grams per hour. Think of it like a supermarket checkout. Glucose alone can only be processed so fast before the gut gets backed up. Fructose opens a second lane, allowing the body to absorb more carbs efficiently. Most good sports nutrition products use this dual-carb approach to maximize fuel delivery without overwhelming the gut.

Sweat Rates and Cramping

Why do some athletes experience cramping, and how can runners prevent it?

Cramping is tricky because it's hard to study. It often happens during races or hard training, making lab conditions unreliable. More recent research shows that cramps aren't always linked to fluid or electrolyte depletion. You see sprinters cramp in a 10-second race or cyclists cramp from a poor bike fit. These are clearly not hydration related.

Dr. Kevin Miller's recent research offers a multifactorial model, suggesting that everyone has a unique "recipe" for cramping. For some, it's electrolyte imbalance. For others, it's fatigue, training errors or biomechanics. Personally, I used to cramp a lot. I sweat heavily, and replacing fluids and sodium helped me.

Tell me more about side aches that runners sometimes experience. What causes them, and how can we prevent them?

It's a common issue, with 15%–25% of runners reporting side stitches in races. There's probably more than one cause, with different types of discomfort often lumped together under "side stitch."

One major factor is timing of food and hydration before running. Many runners notice that eating or drinking too soon before exercise increases their chances of getting a stitch. The first thing to experiment with is adjusting meal timing before workouts.

Some side stitches seem more mechanical. Running involves repetitive impact, and you don't see stitches as often in cycling or swimming. Another theory involves reduced blood flow to the diaphragm and intercostal muscles, especially for newer runners whose breathing muscles aren't fully adapted.

If eating closer to race time is unavoidable, stick to sports drinks, energy gels, or other easily digestible carbs to minimize the risk of discomfort.

There have been major shifts in hydration strategies over the years. What are your thoughts on "drink to thirst" versus structured hydration plans?

Athletes used to be told not to drink at all because it was believed to hinder performance. Then in the '80s, '90s and early 2000s, the message became "Dehydration will ruin your race, so drink as much as you can." Now, we've moved toward "drink to thirst" as a middle ground.

But does drinking to thirst optimize performance? In long or hot races where sweat rates are high, dehydration can develop quickly, and thirst alone might not be the best indicator. When racing under stress, athletes often don't recognize thirst signals until they're already behind. That's why we encourage a blended approach of not sticking to a rigid plan but using guardrails.

For a half-marathon in cool weather, you likely don't need a structured plan. But for a 50K ultra in the summer, having a rough target, like one bottle per hour with a set sodium concentration, provides structure while still allowing adjustments based on how you feel.

The key is finding the balance between listening to your body and having a solid strategy in place.

Can you explain briefly the differences between athletes in terms of sweat rate?

The key difference between athletes is how much sodium they retain. Some people lose as little as 200 milligrams per liter, while others lose over 2,000. I'm on the higher end at about 1,800 milligrams per liter, which is why I get salt rings on my clothes.

The other critical factor is sweat rate. We've tested thousands of athletes, and sweat rates vary wildly. Some lose just 500 milliliters per hour, while others sweat over 3 liters per hour, which is extreme.

What's the best way for athletes to estimate their sweat rate?

The best method is measuring sweat loss directly. Weigh yourself naked before a training session and again after, having toweled off and removed all wet clothing. The difference in weight equals your sweat loss. Doing this test multiple times, in different conditions and workout intensities, gives you a much clearer picture of your hydration needs.

Any final recommendations for athletes wanting to become stronger, healthier and happier?

The biggest takeaway is focusing on four key areas. First, pacing. If I could go back and teach my younger self one thing, it would be how to pace properly. Then, it's about understanding your caloric intake and carbohydrate needs, fluid intake and electrolyte balance. Fuel, hydration and salts are what really matter in endurance performance.

Too often, we get caught up in details like the latest shoes and the best gear, but if your pacing, fueling and hydration aren't dialed in, none of that will save your race. Nail the basics first, then worry about the extras.

Favorite Takeaways from Our YouTube Community

@Ultra-Lawyer – This is one of the best videos I've seen on race nutrition. Best part was the advice with the caveat that everyone is different. Since my ultra journey, I've been focused on eating/drinking while running, but lately, preloading vitamins and minerals such as calcium, potassium and magnesium prevents cramping or real fatigue during the longer training runs. And what I find is, on race day, you default to how well you performed during training, and with a focus on nutrition, the race is more enjoyable. Great content!

@agsmith001 – Thanks for the interesting discussion. I find the discussion on cramps insightful when looking at the other topics from that perspective, i.e., "Everyone has their own personal recipe for cramps," especially with regards to nutrition.

@RobertSmith-God-man – Guys! Thank you so much for sharing. I just ran my second marathon and implemented Andy's advice on fueling. The tip that helped most was taking in fuel during the first part of the race to prepare for the second part. During the last 10 km, the gels tasted awful, but I stuck to the plan, and it helped me finish strong—the first time I'd actually finished all my planned gels! Thanks again.

Kate Martini Freeman on Mindset Coaching

"Push it. Don't decide you can't do something; keep trying. Whether it's a workout, a new distance or whatever it is, it's fun to go after something a little scary. Don't hold back; go for it. Be here, in this moment. Just decide to keep trying. That's where all the magic is. As long as you gave it your best, you'll be stoked."

Kate Martini Freeman was my first running coach, together with her husband, Jimmy Dean Freeman. I've learned a lot from them about hard work, patience and consistency. Her own running journey showcases extraordinary dedication. From finishing her first marathon in just under 5 hours to smashing a personal best of 2:58, Kate transformed herself through years of focused work. Her story goes beyond impressive times. It's about navigating the challenges of training while balancing work, motherhood and staying present in each workout.

Connect:
katemartini.com

Full Episode:
extramilest.com/62

Achieving Consistent Progress

You were able to bring your marathon time from about 5 hours to sub-3. How have you been able to improve over the years?

I wasn't naturally fast, but I loved running. For me, it was all about staying motivated, chipping away at my times, and enjoying the process without stressing over every race. After that first 4:59 marathon, I knew I could do better, and later that same year, I brought it down to 4:24. I just kept training, but the key was making sure I still had fun.

As long as I respected rest days and pulled back when needed, I stayed excited and avoided burnout. In our running group, The Coyotes, we have a saying: "If you're not having fun, you're doing it wrong."

Consistency was everything. I built a strong base that helped me avoid injury and gradually increased mileage. I mixed up my training with different paces, workouts, cross-training and strength work. Especially as a woman, strength training is key for longevity.

Why do you and your husband, Jimmy, incorporate trail running in your coaching approach, even for road runners?

Once we started incorporating trails, we saw our times drop. After a 50-miler (80 km), recovering was often easier because the softer surfaces are gentler on the body. Roads can be brutal. The trails helped not just physically but mentally too. Even when I was chasing a 3:11, 3:09, 3:04 marathon, I still hit the trails, especially in recovery weeks.

Trails give you a different kind of endurance. They also build strength and keep things interesting. Once I incorporated trails regularly, that's when my times dropped. But I'd only take more experienced marathoners to longer distances; for newer runners, I focus more on quality workouts.

In the end, it's about balance. If you've got big goals, go after them, but don't beat your body up unnecessarily. Push hard when needed but listen to your body. Every race teaches you something, and I take those lessons to the next one.

Managing Injuries and the Power of Self-Belief

How do you approach injuries in your training and coaching?

I've had my share of both minor and major injuries. The bigger ones really taught me a lesson because I had to take serious time off from running, which was hard on my ego. It made me realize just how much the body needs real recovery time. I laugh when people say, "I took a week off," like that's enough. Your body doesn't fully heal in a week.

We're so scared to take time off, but how many of us have run through injuries, only to have them linger for months? It's frustrating, but sometimes you need to stop. Talk to your coach, your PT or your doctor.

The key is learning to listen to your body. If something's getting worse mid-run, stop. We've all been there, pushing through pain, but there's a difference between toughing it out and causing long-term damage. It's hard to take time off, but if you give yourself a solid recovery, you'll come back stronger.

What similarities have you seen in athletes who succeed versus those who don't hit their goals?

The one thing that sets successful athletes apart is their belief in themselves. Even if they're not 100% sure, they go for it. They're all in. If you're only halfway committed, it makes everything harder. The people who succeed are the ones who push for something that scares them a little.

The ones who don't reach their goals? It's usually because they're impatient. Big goals take time, sometimes years. Someone who really impacted me was Gordy Ainsleigh, the godfather of ultras. He told me to take a year for each distance increase. Most people aren't patient enough to do that. I wasn't. I jumped from a marathon to a 50-miler (80 km). But I always tell people, go where the inspiration is. If you're excited about something, go for it, but give yourself enough time to train smart.

Do you have any closing thoughts or suggestions for athletes looking to improve?

Be present in the daily process. Honor your body, make adjustments and work on the little things: stability, strength. Push yourself, but don't decide you can't do something before you've tried. Keep going after what's a little scary. That's where the magic happens.

Favorite Takeaways from Our YouTube Community

@ericchevalley – This gem: Check in with your body during your warm-up. Spot on.

@melindachen5462 – As someone who has struggled with injuries, I appreciated the insight around injury prevention—step back weeks, making sure to have a good mileage base before increasing volume—all things I look forward to trying out!

@elizabethdoyle7985 – Don't decide you can't do something. Keep trying. Whether it's a workout or a new distance, it's fun to go after something scary, but then … don't hold back. Don't be afraid to push, and keep pushing.

Matt Fitzgerald on Endurance Mindset

"The best athletes fail a lot because they're setting a high bar. Setting a high bar is also what makes them the best athletes."

Matt Fitzgerald is a lifelong athlete, award-winning endurance sports journalist and bestselling author of more than 20 books, including *80/20 Running, How Bad Do You Want It* and *Running the Dream*. Cofounder of the online training resource 80/20 Endurance, Matt is also an acclaimed endurance coach and nutritionist.

Connect:
mattfitzgerald.org

Full Episodes:
extramilest.com/38
extramilest.com/79

Moderating Training Intensity

Let's talk about the concept of 80/20 running. In your experience, do you see this approach being used by both elite and recreational runners?

The whole 80/20 concept, it's the idea that you should do 80% of your training at low intensity and the other 20% at moderate to high intensity. That's not some scientist's invention. It comes from simply observing elite athletes. That's what they do.

It took a long time to discover it. I don't want to overstate the case. There's no magic in round numbers, but you have to run a lot, and most of your running has to be easy to get the most out of whatever your genetic potential is. So that is what elite athletes do. It's true. You hear the stories, you read the studies, but there's no substitute for direct exposure. That's the reality of it. Elite athletes often run very easy.

Measuring Training Intensity

There are different ways of dialing in your running intensity, besides having to go to a medical lab. What's the best way to figure out easy intensity for the average runner?

The pros really do it by perceived effort. They're very pace-oriented for harder stuff, but for easy runs, it's just by feel. The trouble is, I call it intensity blindness. If I tell the average recreational runner to go out and run for 45 minutes at low intensity, they'll go out and run for 45 minutes at moderate intensity and think it was low intensity.

You need the help of objective metrics: Pace, heart rate and power are the ones that are practically useful in the field. Power is the most reliable in certain ways because a watt is a watt is a watt. Whether you're running with the wind or against the wind, uphill, downhill or on a flat, it's the same number.

Heart rate can be great for holding people back because it's not a performance metric. No one feels compelled to get their heart rate higher.

The talk test is reliable. You can do it anywhere at any time. Stephen Seiler showed that when people exercise just below the ventilatory threshold, they recover much quicker than if they exercised just above it. It really matters.

Mental Resilience Through Injuries

How do you approach running injuries? Any suggestions for staying in a good mental space?

A little exercise I like to give athletes that can help them with that is pretend it's not you. Pretend that the person who got injured is someone you coach. You care about their running, but not the same way. It's like giving relationship advice to a sibling. It is what it is. You cross-train to keep fit. You get a diagnosis. You do corrective exercises to rehab and maybe reduce the likelihood of recurrence.

Pursuing Big Goals

Your book *Running the Dream* was very motivational. Do you have recommendations for athletes looking to set big goals, especially as they age?

One recommendation is don't make any assumptions. If you think something's impossible, just know that you could well be wrong. It's best to assume that you can just keep getting better. Eventually, you won't keep it. Everyone sets their last PR at some point, but I think if you assume, "I can't get better after a certain age," that can become self-fulfilling.

Don't be afraid to fail. When I went to Flagstaff to train at an elite training camp as a recreational runner, I didn't have as much at stake as they did.

Sarah Crouch, a professional runner whom I befriended in Flagstaff, told me, "If you achieve your goals more than 50% of the time, you need to raise the bar." It's okay to fail. The best athletes fail a lot because they're setting a high bar. Setting a high bar is also what makes them the best athletes.

Any closing advice to become a stronger, happier and healthier athlete?

One thing I was able to bring home with me from my elite training camp experience was the professionals' no-stone-unturned mindset. When your very livelihood depends on your performance, you don't just say, "Oh, bad luck." When something goes wrong, you try to figure it out. You try to get an answer. You try to do what you can.

Favorite Takeaways from Our YouTube Community

@DanielL143 – What you said about staying rational, objective and detaching from yourself as though you were coaching someone else. Matt, this is pure gold. I just did a crappy 5-mile (8 km) run and felt down and convinced myself that I should give up running, then I forced myself to do the same route the next day and felt fantastic.

@MrsChristie76 – My takeaway is Matt's suggestion of going for a goal that is way above your comfort levels with a 10% chance of achieving. Even if you fail, you win!

@nicholashernandez6060 – The idea of reframing/renaming "my injured knee" to "my healing knee." I think this can be very useful to someone like me who sometimes speaks in a slightly pessimistic way.

@dsfrye01 – I really like Matt's comment of "Everything is figure-outable." It's so true. When we get away from the emotional state we are in, things can get better. So many wonderful nuggets. Pain is a signal. It doesn't have to be a stop sign.

Kyle Long on Strength Training

"Have goals throughout the year that you're building toward, whether it's a race or a self-guided project. Take time to plan how you'll achieve those goals. Having structure, whether through a run coach or a specific program, makes the training journey more enjoyable and effective."

Kyle Long is a seasoned strength, conditioning and run coach with a strong background in ultra-endurance sports. Known for his powerful, practical approach, he has helped countless athletes strengthen traditionally weak areas to boost running performance. Based in the Pacific Northwest, Kyle embraces the rugged terrain, often taking on volcanic landscapes to train both body and mind.

Connect:
instagram.com/100milekyle

Full Episode:
extramilest.com/81

Structured Weight Training

How can runners implement strength training consistently and actually stick with it?

One of the biggest problems with implementing strength work into a run program is twofold. First, people often jump in at such an intensity level that it starts to negatively impact their run performance. After the initial excitement wears off, they notice their run performance drops because they're training too hard in the gym, not using it as an accessory to improve their running.

Second, most people just bounce around between what I call the "sexy exercises" without following a steady, progressive build over six to eight months. The workouts really shouldn't look that different over a four-, six- or eight-week block; they should be progressive in terms of weight, reps and movement intensity. Having a structured program over a six- to eight-week plan helps you stick to it more, just like a running plan.

If you're new to strength training, the first few days will beat you up a bit, even if the intensity is about right. But beyond that, my rule for runners is that your strength work should never negatively impact your priority runs. It should always be a positive part of your week in terms of performance.

What about busy people who find it difficult to fit in multiple strength sessions in a week?

I'd rather athletes stack strength work on days they are doing big efforts outdoors than sprinkling them in between. Your body is primed, and even if you've gone out for a lot of miles, it's better to stack strength work after a long or hard effort. This way, you don't end up with every other day being a hard day, allowing you to have some true recovery days.

Avoiding Pitfalls

What are some common mistakes runners make around strength training?

The most common mistake is not progressing a program. They might go to the gym two or three times a week for 30–45 minutes, but if you zoom out over two months, there's no steady linear progression. If you've been back-squatting for six weeks, you might switch to front squats for the next block. This keeps the workouts fresh while continuing to build strength.

What's the minimum equipment needed for strength training? Can you get away with bodyweight exercises only?

If you're setting up a home program, think about moving horizontally and vertically. For upper and lower body, push and pull, you can do a lot with minimal equipment: bodyweight exercises like squats, lunges, pushups and pull-ups. If you're new to strength work, a bodyweight program is sufficient. As you progress, adding resistance bands, a few kettlebells, or dumbbells up to 25 pounds (11 kg) can be beneficial. These can cover most of what you need without the complexity of advanced strength work.

What would be a simple workout that anyone can find time for say, 10–15 minutes, that can still make a gain in strength?

For a quick workout, I recommend an upper body push, upper body pull, lower body push and lower body pull. For example, pushups, pull-ups, bodyweight squats and glute bridges. Cycle through these exercises for 12 minutes, doing as many rounds as you can. It's efficient, effective and requires no equipment.

You can find some of Kyle Long's follow-along workouts at extramilest.com/kylelong.

Jason Fitzgerald on Injury Prevention

"Most injuries are because of the three too's: too much, too soon, too fast. So, you're doing too much mileage too soon before you're ready for it, and you're probably running some of it too fast."

Jason Fitzgerald is a running coach, bestselling author and host of *The Strength Running Podcast*. Having battled through his own share of running injuries as a collegiate athlete, Jason transformed his struggles into expertise, becoming a trusted voice in injury prevention for runners.

Connect:
instagram.com/jasonfitz1

Full Episode:
extramilest.com/103

Minimizing Running-Related Injuries

How can runners identify when it's time to back off from training to avoid injury?

I have a simple three-step check-in method:

- **Pain Type:** Sharp, stabbing pains are a red flag. Dull, achy discomfort might be manageable.
- **Pain Progression:** If the discomfort gets worse as you run, stop. It's probably worsening the injury.
- **Running Form:** If pain alters your running gait or causes compensations, that's another clear sign you should stop. Continuing will lead to additional problems.

What strength and mobility exercises do you recommend most for runners to prevent injuries?

I'm fairly exercise agnostic. Consistency with a structured routine matters more than specific moves. But fundamental exercises I recommend include bridges, side-lying leg raises, clamshells, planks, squats, deadlifts, lunges and side planks. Routines built around these movements help runners maintain good form, improve overall athleticism and significantly reduce injury risk.

What affordable strength and mobility tools would you suggest for recreational runners?

Some versatile, affordable tools I highly recommend are:

- **Resistance bands:** Great for lateral walks, monster walks, clamshells and leg raises.
- **Kettlebells:** Extremely versatile for strength and explosive movements. Beginners should start at around 15–20 lbs.
- **Foam rollers:** Excellent for interactive muscle exploration, improving mobility and identifying imbalances.

Do you have any mental advice for runners dealing with injuries?

The best psychological approach to injury is to attack your recovery with the same enthusiasm as your regular training. If you can't run, there's still plenty you can do: physical therapy, mobility work, pool running. Treat these as your training for now. Recognizing injuries as part of the running journey and maintaining active involvement in your recovery helps manage the mental challenges and preserves your identity as an athlete.

> ### Favorite Takeaways From Our YouTube Community
>
> **@rickj6594 -** My favorite part is the reminder that running is not just running. Sleep, strength, yoga, flexibility, etc all support running.
>
> **@erikthiel279 -** Too much, too soon, too fast. Ill remember this forever. I'm signed up for my first marathon in October and I'm already dealing with early stages of shin splints. I def got excited and fell victim to the 3 too's. Ill hit the stationary bike and hope i got time to heal, train, and make it to the start line.
>
> **@the_humble_runner -** Absolutely amazing episode Floris! Being injured now for 6 months with Plantar Fasciitis, this is like a breath of fresh air ... I will continue to be attacking my recovery and rehabilitation with the same intensity and discipline like a regular training for marathons ... I am just taking a detour to my final destination.
>
> **@liljemark1 -** Your discussion around being an athlete who specializes in running was a good one. As I've almost hit age 45 I've realized muscle mass is not easy to gain or keep so I want to do my best to stay strong, and see how it helps my running. A small home gym has been a lifesaver when there's small kids in the family and difficult to find time for myself.

Dr. Mark Cucuzzella on Healthy Running

"Yeah, I progressed from an 11-minute mile (6:50 min/km) at a heart rate of 152 to pretty close to a 6-ish-minute mile (3:44 min/km) over the course of four months. If you finish a training run and you don't think you could do that again, you've probably trained too hard."

Dr. Mark Cucuzzella is a physician and professor of family medicine at West Virginia University School of Medicine. He's also been a runner for more than three decades, with a personal best of 2:24 in the marathon. He's run the Boston Marathon 25 times and previously held the record for the longest streak of sub-3-hour marathon finishes: 30 years! He is also deeply involved in designing injury-reduction programs for military personnel, owns a minimalist footwear store and is a race director and author.

Connect:
drmarksdesk.com

Full Episodes:
extramilest.com/18
extramilest.com/58

Low Heart Rate Fundamentals

How did you first discover low heart rate training and what happened when you tried it?

I first discovered the Maffetone Method on a United Airlines flight, reading an article by Mark Allen titled something like "Get Fast, Run Slow." It changed my life. Allen had lost six Ironman titles to Dave Scott, then started training with Phil Maffetone, using the 180-minus-age formula to keep his heart rate low. Inspired, I bought a $50 heart rate monitor, and even though I was jogging at an 11-minute/mile pace (6:50 min/km) while others passed me, I trusted the process.

Over four months, I went from running an 11-minute mile (6:50/km) at a 152 heart rate to a 6-minute mile (3:44/km). That fall, I was unexpectedly called to run the Marine Corps Marathon. Despite no race prep, I hit the halfway mark at 1:15 and finished feeling like I could run it again. It was an incredible result from low heart rate training.

It's hard for Type A runners to slow down, but pushing constantly can break you, as many runners with cardiac issues can attest. Training shouldn't leave you exhausted; even Eliud Kipchoge rarely goes beyond 80% in training. If you finish a training run and you don't think you could do that again, you're probably training too hard.

I see it over and over again with people just starting out, when they have to slow down. You slow down your time and you feel like you have to leave your pride at the door. A lot of people who are a lot slower than you will be passing you left and right. You just have to accept that this is the case in training, at the beginning. But over time, and pretty quickly if things line up, you start to speed up and everything changes from there.

What advice would you give to someone starting low heart rate training who might struggle with progress?

Choosing the right heart rate is key. Most people haven't been to an exercise lab, which would be ideal for pinpointing their zone, so we rely on guidelines. Here's a simple indicator: When we burn glucose, we produce more carbon dioxide, but when we burn fat, we produce less. In the lab, we call this "respiratory exchange ratio." Ideally, you're using fat as fuel at easier paces, while harder efforts shift you to glucose burning. A good sign you're in the right zone is if you can still carry on a conversation.

But there's more to it than just effort. Factors like sleep, stress and diet can all impact performance. If someone's sleep deprived, under family stress or eating poorly, they're going to have a tough time improving, even with the right heart rate.

It's crucial to remember that training is highly individual. High-volume training works for some but not others, depending on factors like muscle fiber type. Working with a coach or advisor helps, as they can spot underlying issues. Sometimes, a medical condition like anemia or thyroid imbalance could be the culprit, or life might just be too full. Think Ironman training on four hours of sleep with two full-time jobs.

A Moving Meditation

What advice would you give athletes looking to improve their race times while becoming stronger, healthier and happier?

I think what's between your ears is the biggest factor. You've got to be having fun. If you're not waking up excited to get outside, then it's time to check in. What's going on? Are you sleep deprived, stressed? Running should add time to your day, not take it away. When you're out there, it should feel like a moving meditation, ideally out in the sunlight. Running shouldn't be another stress in your life because that'll backfire.

For me, running is recovery from life, so every day is a recovery run. Life is busy and full with kids, work, so if running didn't recharge me, it'd be hard to keep up. That's the takeaway: Let running be your recovery. Some days, you'll feel incredible and run fast, like you're flying. Other days, you're just out there, taking it slow; breathing, maybe even running barefoot. It's got to stay enjoyable. If you wake up and don't feel like running, take a day off and see what's up.

Heart rate also tells you a lot about your physiology and metabolism. It shows how you're accessing fuel; how you're teaching your body to burn fat efficiently. Mark Allen was doing this before "fat max" was even a known term. Fat max is your sweet spot—the fastest pace at which you're optimizing fat burning. Push harder than that, and you start "burning matches," tapping into limited resources.

What are your thoughts on stretching and mobility?

First, you need to assess your own mobility. If you're in good shape, you don't necessarily need to stretch. Just maintain what you've got. There's a balance; too much mobility isn't good because it can make you unstable. The hips are usually where people are tight, especially from sitting.

Movements like walking lunges help open up the hips. Even at work, you can make adjustments. If you're at a corporate meeting, sit on the edge of the chair with one leg back to open up your hip, then switch sides after a while.

I also use foam rolling daily, especially on the hip flexors. The hip capsule stiffens as we age. If nothing else, focus on your hips. Don't sit all day, and keep them open.

Community Improves Health and Longevity

Blue Zones are regions where people live exceptionally long lives. How do factors like community and purpose contribute to health and running performance?

Through observational research, we examine cohorts of people who live long and healthy lives. One of the most robust datasets is the *Baltimore Longitudinal Study of Aging* (National Institute on Aging; last accessed online, July 20, 2025, https://www.blsa.nih.gov/).

Loneliness is deadly. When people feel lonely, it's extremely toxic, triggering different neurochemical signals.

Having a purpose is crucial. The study found that one of the most important indicators of longevity is having a sense of purpose. People with a purpose rarely fully retire; they're always engaged in something meaningful. Although it's hard to measure objectively, this factor stands out as more significant than cholesterol levels or genetic makeup. This purpose can come from various sources, such as a church community. Tight-knit church communities thrive because members receive social and emotional support, and a sense of purpose.

Giving back is also essential. When people donate to charity anonymously, whether it's their time or money, they do so without expecting anything in return. This selfless giving positively impacts their health, something we don't see as much in modern, capitalistic societies.

Many readers are looking to improve their running and overall health. What final thoughts would you share with them?

It's basic: Eat like a human—eat real food; move gently and easily without pain. Fit running into your life. When you come back from a run, you should feel better. This should add to your day, not be like another chore. I run in the morning; I'm a little stiff, but I've never not felt better at the end of a run than when I went out the door. So if the opposite is happening to you, you're doing something wrong. You should always feel better when you come back, and you should wake up tomorrow, maybe it's a day you just don't have time, but you should always feel, oh man, I could run today, right? I feel good, I could run today.

If you really don't feel like running, something's wrong either in your health or your running or your life or your mood. Running is such a powerful mood enhancer. If running isn't making you happy, something is really jacked up in your life somewhere. Talk to someone who can help you, right? Because this could be one of many things; you really need someone who can look at you medically and even spiritually. We're not just a bunch of parts.

Favorite Takeaways from Our YouTube Community

@pradeepkumarka – The best conclusion I got from Dr. Cucuzzella's closing comments: One should feel better and energetic after a workout. As always you are doing a great service to the running community, Floris.

@Rls2236 – I love hearing Mark talking about how the elite runners take the majority of their runs super easy and save the special workouts and special shoes for a small percentage of their overall running. It's a good lesson for everyone.

@titosinha – "Finish every workout with a smile." Thank you so much, Floris, for such an illuminating discussion with Dr. Cucuzzella. The approaches you've laid out in your program and explored with your guests have been life transforming for me.

@franciscomontoya92 – "If you finish the workout and don't feel that you can do it again right away, you're probably training too hard." This is great advice!!

@evanjamison8907 – What I took away was the necessity of fun. I often see running as a chore or, worse, a perpetual competition. Gotta check that ego and run for the pure joy of it.

Matteo Franceschetti on Sleep Optimization

"Sleep is foundational to your overall performance, and we refer to it as 'sleep fitness.' Approach sleep with the same mindset you apply to daily training. Dedicate the necessary time and prioritize it. Doing so will reflect in your biometrics, boost your energy and improve your athletic performance."

Matteo Franceschetti is the cofounder and CEO of Eight Sleep, a company making waves in the athletic world through sleep technology. Matteo helps athletes optimize their recovery with Eight Sleep's temperature-regulating "Pod" system. His innovative approach to sleep as a performance tool has earned recognition from *Time* and *Fast Company*, with athletes now using his technology to boost recovery and performance.

Connect:
matteofranceschetti.com

Full Episode:
extramilest.com/87

Sleep Is a Key Pillar of Health

You have talked about using sleep as a competitive advantage, not just in your actual training but also in professional and personal life. Can you explain that further?

Sleep is one of the three pillars of health: sleep, nutrition and fitness, and it actually comes first. If you're not sleeping well, it affects everything. You start craving junk food, you don't feel like training, and your performance drops. Treat sleep like you do your training, putting in the time and consistency, and you'll see it reflected in your biometrics, energy and overall performance.

What are common sleep mistakes that you're seeing among athletes?

The biggest issues are inconsistent bedtimes and not getting enough sleep. People often confuse their body's natural rhythm by going to bed and waking up at different times, which can feel like switching time zones. Alcohol and heavy meals before bed are also common mistakes. They negatively impact your sleep quality. Another big one is a racing mind. People can't calm down before bed, which leads to poor sleep.

What are your thoughts on naps? Can you take an optimal nap that can actually benefit you?

I'm a huge supporter of naps! They can be a performance enhancer if done right. The key is to keep them short, about 20–30 minutes, so you don't get into deep sleep or REM. I also recommend a "napuccino," where you drink a coffee right before your nap. The caffeine kicks in after 30 minutes, just as you're waking up, so you feel supercharged.

Improving Sleep Fitness

Why do you think so many people still struggle with maintaining consistent high-quality sleep even when they prioritize it?

We call it "sleep fitness" at Eight Sleep because, just like fitness, sleep requires effort. A lot of people don't put the same preparation into sleep as they would into a workout. Plus, we've conditioned ourselves to think that sleep isn't as important, even though it's foundational. Also, people don't have a solid bedtime routine, so their body doesn't know it's time to wind down. And if your mind is racing, that can be a big barrier to falling asleep.

How much sleep do you need if you're training more than five hours a week?

Athletes should aim for eight to nine hours of sleep a night. The more they sleep, the better, especially to reduce the risk of injury. If they've had a tough workout, I'd also recommend a nap afterward to help with recovery.

Removing Obstacles to Sleep

How would you go about trying to increase your time sleeping?

If you have trouble falling or staying asleep, I'd suggest doing some research on cognitive behavioral therapy for insomnia (CBTI). It's important not to spend too much time in bed awake, as your brain can associate the bed with not sleeping, creating anxiety. If you're struggling with sleep, try compressing your sleep window to make yourself more tired. Avoid napping if it affects your nighttime sleep, and focus on establishing a consistent sleep routine.

Favorite Takeaways from Our YouTube Community

@jessewu7040 – "Sleep fitness"—having the same mindset for sleep as athletes have for working out! Thanks for this broadcast; it is something that needs attention in my life.

@skalnik94able – Sleep is the top priority in your training! Thank you for that well-needed reminder!

@avraver12 – The tip on adjusting LED lights to warm before bedtime. I usually get about 6 hours of sleep, trying to get 7 ideally.

Kara Collier on Glucose Management

"Prioritize starting your meal with protein, especially before consuming carbohydrates. This helps keep blood sugar levels more stable."

Kara Collier, RDN, LDN, CNSC, is the cofounder and VP of health at Nutrisense, a wellness startup specializing in personalized health monitoring. A *Forbes* 30 Under 30 recipient, Kara uses continuous glucose monitoring (CGM) technology to help nondiabetics optimize health and prevent metabolic diseases. With a clinical nutrition background, she pairs modern technology with expert coaching to improve glucose control and longevity.

Connect:
karacollier.com

Full Episode:
extramilest.com/53

Balancing Glucose for Steady Energy

How are glucose levels and energy levels correlated?

They're tightly correlated. When our glucose swings up and down throughout the day, it often results in our feeling drained or fatigued. The more we can even out glucose levels, the better we'll typically feel. Reactive hypoglycemia, where glucose spikes and then crashes, is more common than documented. It usually leads to fatigue, post-meal slumps or cravings, starting a vicious cycle.

What can we do to stabilize blood sugar levels or minimize big swings?

When optimizing glucose values, think about the four pillars of glucose control.

- The first pillar is nutrition. Meal spikes can be minimized by experimenting with different strategies.
- The second pillar is physical activity, focusing on increasing physical fitness, adding lean body mass and increasing daily movement.
- The third pillar is stress management.
- The fourth pillar is sleep. Stress and sleep are equally important and should be prioritized alongside exercise and diet.

Nutrition and Fueling Strategies

What are some key lessons you've found regarding nutrition?

A key takeaway is to avoid "naked carbs." Try not to eat carbohydrates alone. Start your meal with protein and some fat before consuming carbs. Another key is carbohydrate processing. The more processed a carbohydrate is, the more dramatic the glucose response. For example, steel-cut oats will have a lower glucose response compared to instant oats. The form of food, liquid versus solid, also matters. Focus on real food as much as possible and be mindful of meal timing. Eating earlier in the day often results in lower glucose responses than eating the same meal later.

What about intermittent fasting or snacking throughout the day?

It depends on your goals. As a general rule, try to fast for 12 to 14 hours, avoid food at least 3 hours before bed and avoid constant grazing. Grazing can lead to minor glucose peaks all day, which raises your overall average.

However, for athletes with high energy demands, underfueling is often an issue. If someone is undereating, it's better to eat four to six meals rather than focusing too much on intermittent fasting. For those with insulin resistance, fasting can be an effective tool, but it's all about context.

Optimizing Physical Activity

What are some findings related to physical activity and glucose control?

Physical activity significantly improves glucose control. We think about it through three components: endurance activity, lean body mass and movement throughout the day. Endurance training helps, but adding lean body mass is crucial as muscles are the largest sink for glucose. Gentle movement, like a 10- to 15-minute walk after meals, can also help blunt glucose responses.

Any closing thoughts for recreational runners to become stronger, healthier and happier athletes?

Focus on fueling properly. Track your calorie and protein intake and ensure you're giving your body what it needs to perform at its best. Awareness, tracking and adjusting based on data are key.

Favorite Takeaways from Our YouTube Community

@kenklee4 – I love the idea of eating the proteins before carbs. So fascinating that something so simple can have good effects.

@mpvsystems9302 – Probably the most counterintuitive findings I have learned from the CGM is that Zone 2 aerobic training drives my blood glucose down and anaerobic workouts drive it up.

@ameliavrabel2125 – I think the biggest takeaway here that many athletes are guilty of is not to "do your workout" or "get your 10,000 steps" and then be sedentary the rest of the day. This is one thing I do like about how my watch reminds me to move every hour or it is easy to get stuck in a chair or on the couch.

Tawnee Prazak Gibson on Holistic Health

"What's tricky with endurance sports is that we can see a very clear crossover between good athlete traits and traits of those with eating disorders. They all sound like great things, right? We want to see somebody who's mentally tough, committed, pursuing excellence and willing to push through pain. However, all of those things have a direct tie-in with what constitutes somebody suffering greatly from an eating disorder. So it gets really tricky."

Tawnee Prazak Gibson is a holistic health and endurance sports coach, known for competing in the Boston Marathon and Ironman 70.3 World Championships. Having overcome disordered eating and exercise addiction, she now educates athletes on the importance of balance, self-care and community support for health and success. Her approach to training and nutrition is holistic, emphasizing flexibility, gut health and listening to the body's needs rather than adhering strictly to rigid diets.

Connect:
instagram.com/tawneegibson

Full Episode:
extramilest.com/42

Healthy Eating vs. Disordered Eating

What are common disordered eating habits you're seeing among athletes?

Anorexia and bulimia are some of the worst, and they're relatively clear diagnosable conditions. But now we have this spectrum of disordered eating patterns, where someone isn't clinically diagnosed but is subclinically suffering from an unhealthy relationship with food, body and exercise. They're fixated on unhealthy habits, the need for control, perfectionism in diet, and can't waver from certain rules. For example, people with orthorexia who cancel dinner plans because the restaurant doesn't serve organic food or uses canola oil instead of olive oil. It's okay to talk about a healthy diet, but the key is not being overly rigid where it controls your whole life.

It's upon ourselves to dive inward and ask hard questions. Are we honoring our body's true needs? When you find disordered patterns, if you're being honest, you know deep down you've veered away from serving your best well-being. You're stuck in a mindset that you can't break free from, and you feel guilt and shame because you're not honoring your true needs.

It's hard to define because it manifests differently in people. Today, you have one doctor saying intermittent fasting is the best thing ever and another saying don't touch it with a 10-foot pole. It can be overwhelming, so I completely empathize with people feeling frozen and unsure of what to do.

Athletes sometimes assume intermittent fasting is the be-all and end-all answer to a healthy life. But if your body isn't functioning properly, fasting might add additional stress. An individualized approach is crucial. What's your perspective?

Exactly. For example, I've been presented with chronically high cortisol in the morning, yet I used to do fasted runs and drink coffee on an empty stomach, believing it would help develop metabolic efficiency. It seemed fine until I realized it was screwing up my health.

Now, I refuse to run fasted in the morning or drink coffee on an empty stomach. I still like to work out in the morning, but I find it's better for me to work out in the afternoons when my cortisol is more balanced.

I see this a lot in endurance athletes, especially female clients who fast before runs to avoid gut distress. But fasting every run, especially long or double days, is a fast track to damaging your well-being. We have to dive into gut health and address underlying issues.

Common Fueling Mistakes

What are common nutritional deficiencies among athletes?

The #1 deficiency I see is protein intake. Athletes often aren't fueling enough for their caloric expenditure, leading to underfueling in general. Protein intake, in particular, tends to be low. Research shows we can safely consume up to 2 grams per kilogram of body weight, but most find it hard to get that amount.

We also see deficiencies like vitamin D, B12 and iron, but I try to look at the full picture. Sometimes, deficiencies are related to gut health issues rather than diet alone. Athletes may eat a well-rounded diet but still be deficient due to gut dysfunction, which requires diving into the root cause and pursuing healing.

Training for Long-Term Health

How has your training approach changed over time?

Back then, I had this thing in my head where I had to accumulate eight hours of training by Friday. It was nonnegotiable, and I wouldn't budge—even through injury or fatigue. I was relentless in pursuing perfection, and it left no room for listening to my body or emotions.

These days, I'm much more relaxed in my approach. I've learned to honor my body's needs in whatever season I'm in. For example, during pregnancy, I embraced the changes in my body and laughed at myself when hobbling around a track at a 12-minute-per-mile pace (7:27 min/km). It was about feeling good and celebrating small victories rather than being fixated on big goals.

I've had athletes where we've mutually decided to take a step back from training because of life circumstances. It's okay to say that a goal needs to be put on the shelf for a while. Honoring our well-being is so important, and it's okay to adjust priorities. The races will be there again when the time is right.

How did your journey overcoming disordered eating impact your approach?

When you push your body to extremes without care, you burn out. Sure, I qualified for championships, but it was short-lived. My stress balance was way out of whack, with mood disturbances, epic breakdowns, horrible gut health and amenorrhea for a decade. Eventually, it ate away at me, especially as I became a voice in endurance sports while being dysfunctional myself. My performance tanked. I had to start addressing what was happening mentally and physically, completely shifting my training and career.

Any advice for athletes to become healthier, happier and stronger?

Sleep and rest. Don't deny your body the recovery it needs. You are human, and you need to recover. Get seven to eight hours of sleep a night. Your athletic performance will suffer if you don't.

Favorite Takeaways from Our YouTube Community

@burillakcsaba – My takeaway is to trust the process and don't be afraid whether you reach your goal at the end. That's a big one. If you believe in what you are doing, being afraid of the end result might just undermine success.

@serenasbeauty – Listen to your body. Put goals on hold. Every winter I have to do this because I teach, and when I up my running, I become too stressed to be good to my students and my own kids. Summer training for fall races is my new plan.

@KiranKMeka – Slow down, trust the process, support network of friends, honoring yourself, less stress. So many important points that one can implement in daily life to improve holistically.

Chris Hauth on Mental Toughness

"The gradual approach allows you to figure out your deeper why. After about six weeks the doldrums come, where life starts getting in the way, fatigue accumulates, and it gets hard. It's not about being a role model for your kids; they're not awake to see you get out the door. It's about your own deeper internal reason why."

Chris Hauth pushes the limits of human endurance as a two-time Olympian and ultra-athlete who's built a life around going further and digging deeper. After starting as an Olympic swimmer, Chris found his groove in triathlons and ultrarunning, where he discovered that physical challenges reveal who we truly are. He completed seven marathons on seven continents in seven days, showing firsthand that when things get tough, that's when we learn the most about ourselves.

Connect:
instagram.com/AIMPCoach

Full Episode:
extramilest.com/66

Let's say you're looking to level up from a 5K to a 10K, or from a half-marathon to a full marathon. What advice do you have for runners entering new, intimidating territory?

I always look for curiosity first. If the athlete is curious about what's on the other side of that finish line, that's powerful. When you expand your endurance, you're discovering more about yourself. You're going on a quest, not only on race day but through all the training leading up to it. Whether it's a 30-minute run or a 2-hour run, it's time to yourself, in your head. It's mental and physical growth simultaneously.

You talk about "working in" versus "working out." Can you explain that concept?

Many think about working out as something physical, looking better, losing weight. But in endurance, you have an opportunity to work in, to develop self-growth and awareness. It's like meditation; a daily check-in with yourself.

As distances get longer, it becomes less a physical question and more mental. How do I manage my emotions and thoughts to continue moving forward? We all have the monkey mind with negative chatter swirling around. Mental fortitude is a muscle that can be trained, just like a physical one. The more reps we have talking to that voice, the better we get at handling it.

How do you view failure and setting big, scary goals?

If you know you can do something, you won't apply all your faculties to it. It doesn't bring forth your best effort. I think fear is a huge component of setting big, audacious goals. That fear sits on the wall between your current reality and the opportunity on the other side.

When you're stripped raw emotionally and physically in a challenge, what version of you comes forward? There's something magical there. You learn so much about yourself and get a glimpse of who you actually are. That's what makes the achievement meaningful.

What's your most important advice for athletes looking to improve?

Consistency over time is the key to endurance. Even a 15-minute run or walk, done consistently, creates an engine. Your intentional showing up over time makes a huge difference.

Longevity and consistency are superpowers. There might be faster or stronger athletes, but if you stay in the arena long enough, you'll whittle down the field. You'll look back in six months and realize how far you've come. It doesn't need to be huge steps. It's progress over time. That's growth: consistency over time.

Favorite Takeaways from Our YouTube Community

@WendyRedeemed – Appreciated the "working in" rather than just "working out." Learning to observe how we react in adversity and developing mental toughness to manage negative emotions and thoughts is powerful. We truly find out who we are in those tough moments.

@CODxClIpZ – Nothing matters more than long-term consistency. Consistently small efforts trump occasionally great efforts. You can take a microstep toward your fitness and endurance right now. It doesn't have to be a 60-minute run; go run for 10 minutes. Injured? Go walk for 10 minutes. Start small and stay consistent.

@morrisg5060 – Being curious about what my body can accomplish is such an adventure. My biggest takeaway: We can achieve more than we think if we give it time and build up safely. I'm signed up for a 50K ultra in Moab, Utah, without ever running a marathon. It's a little crazy at 46, but I'm excited for the journey!

@toddmarentette – Love this podcast, advice and message. "Longevity and consistency wins" … Chris is right on. There will always be faster, stronger ones. That's not what it's about. The conversation about being prepared for the down that comes after a big adventure is impactful. Keep it weird!

Jimmy Dean Freeman on Mental Training

"The wall isn't there to stop you from your dream. The wall is there to see how bad you want it. You have to be able to roll with the punches. You have to be able to follow your dream. If it were easy, everyone would do it and it wouldn't be as meaningful, so the wall is there to test how much you want it."

Jimmy Dean Freeman is the head coach and founder of Coyote Running, with nearly four decades of competitive running experience spanning over 200 races. Known for his expertise in mental training, Jimmy has coached more than 2,000 athletes since 2002, helping them break through self-imposed limitations. His personal accomplishments include the Boston Marathon, Western States 100, Angeles Crest 100 and the grueling Badwater 135, with impressive personal bests of 2:56 in the marathon and 17:34 in the 100-miler (161 km). Jimmy and his wife, Kate Martini Freeman, help athletes focus on process over outcome, teaching them to stay present in each moment.

Connect:
instagram.com/coachjimmydean

Full Episode:
extramilest.com/59

Getting Your Mental Process Right

I've heard you talk numerous times about training your mind and about a glass ceiling that you can push and move further. Can you talk about that more?

Yeah, I think people get really focused on "I have a goal," and let's say the goal is to qualify for the Boston Marathon. There's a time associated with that for my age and gender, and whatever that is—a common goal in the running world, or to break 4 hours in a marathon or to break 3 hours—whatever it is. We start by seeking information about what workouts we need to do to make that happen.

One of the main elements of this experience and how to really drive the most out of your body is your mental process. How are you thinking about it, both in training and during the race? Now, the glass ceiling in this particular realm is a level of achievement we think we're personally capable of. We all have some idea of "I think I could do this."

The glass ceiling idea is that we all have an idea of the lid on our peak performance. To be honest, we don't know. Science doesn't know. We can project. But what if you were to live and train with that as a question mark instead of knowing what you think you're capable of, just giving up the idea that you have any idea, and saying, "I'm going to treat this as an adventure, as an exploration, and see"?

For me, that question manifested in running the Badwater 135-mile (217 km) race. It manifested in running the Original Six Hundo Challenge, doing the six original 100-milers (161 km) inside of 13 weeks. I didn't know if I could do that. I didn't really believe one way or another. I just went for it. This summer, I'm going to live the question. It's not about achieving it or not. It's about what quality your life takes on when you're in the space of adventurous inquiry. You're either living on the edge, living a daring life, or you're wasting it.

When you look at all the different athletes you've coached, you see some aiming high and reaching their goals while others miss their goals. What are some general characteristics between people who reach their goal, and those who don't reach what they set out to do?

There are two major factors that play a part in goal achievement. One element, at least in our sport, is a genetic predisposition. You have a baseline VO_2 max.

How well your body produces, processes and utilizes oxygen is a big factor in long-distance running. Another factor is physical durability. Some people can handle very stressful workouts and recover from them quickly. When we're younger, we can bounce back more quickly. Each individual person's body type—their biomechanics—leads to less injury or more injury. Some people's bones and tendons hold up better than others. It's just the nature of the game.

There's also the mental side. Some people have the disposition to go very hyperbolic. In our day and age, people are really impatient. I see more people signing up for a running program having never done a marathon, already talking about a 100-miler (161 km) this year. Then there are other people who have been running marathons for 15 years and just want to run five minutes faster.

I think there's a long game that we need to play. You want to pick a goal that will take five or more years to achieve; something that you can't even imagine yourself doing right now. The process of exploration, discovery and perseverance you'll go through to get there will put your life into a very distinct space in the day-to-day of chasing after that. The idea that "I'm going to set this goal, and I better achieve it this year or I'm done," and people who get injured and quit right away, "Oh, this just isn't meant for me," that's the main thing.

You once told me before my first sub-3 marathon that I might feel a 2/10 discomfort that could quickly escalate to a 9/10. How important is it to avoid going into a race overconfident?

Yeah, I've had this happen a number of times in 100-mile (161-km) races. Don't count your chickens before they're hatched. When you're at mile 16 (26 km) and feeling great, you're like, "I feel better than I've ever felt at any mile 16." And then, at mile 17 (27 km), sh*t hits the fan. Being sort of mentally and emotionally nimble will allow for the nonlinear experience to happen.

From my perspective, those who get good at that flow in their races, long-distance races and training sessions, find a way to apply that to their lives. Life is about as nonlinear as it gets. One month you're on top of your bills and your savings, doing great, and then the next month some tragedy happens and throws things sideways for a while. Learning to deal with whatever comes up, it just comes back to a little saying that I say to myself: "What can I do right now?"

For some races, I write the letters on my hand: WCIDRN, which stands for "What can I do right now?" The idea is, whether things are going great or bad, what can I do right now to make the next moment better? What can I do right now to make the next hour better? What can I do right now to make this race better? It gets you present again, and then it's not about what's gone wrong, because we can sometimes get focused on the negative. It's "What can I do to move through this?"

A lot of these lessons apply to training, racing and life.

Big time. I think sometimes people get so hyper-focused on race day when really, for the sake of argument, it's six months of training leading into it. If you can survive that and get to the race healthy enough, fit enough and motivated enough, you're 90% of the way there. Race day is critical. You have to execute on race day. There's no faking fitness. If you're fit enough, you can do it. If you don't hit the time, it doesn't mean you weren't fit enough. But surviving the training block is an even bigger piece than how you execute the race, but both count.

Do you have any recommendations for athletes to become stronger, healthier and happier?

A lot of what we do in the early stages of our running is guesswork. My attitude toward running is that it's an experiential sport, and we're going to learn the lessons by making the mistakes ourselves. Accountability is a big piece of it. Accountability structures can show up in your life in a number of ways. You can hire a coach, sign up for a training program like the Personal Best Program, go to a running club and have a regular run with people where you're all engaged in sharing your goals with each other. It can be something you share with your spouse. Having a defined set of goals and a timeline gives you that map to accountability. If there isn't a set goal—if there isn't someone to hold you accountable outside of yourself—the snooze button looms large. The "I can do it tomorrow" mentality creeps in.

Favorite Takeaways from Our YouTube Community

@hobyr3439 – "Dream Big." That's it. Sometimes life gets in the way, but today I got reminded again to believe in them.

@jeffmacpherson4283 – "We all have an idea of what the lid is on our peak performance. We can project, but if you were to live and train with that as a question mark, instead of 'knowing' what you think you're capable of; just giving up the idea that you have any idea and saying, 'I'm going to treat this as an adventure …'"

@sigfreed11 – I really appreciated that he talked about running isn't all about pace and physical improvement but rather mental and emotional improvement outside of running.

@4tomansky – My favorite quote of this awesome episode is: "The wall isn't there to stop you from your dream; the wall is there to see how bad you want it." That one hits hard!

@rorymurphy3975 – As a "restart" runner at the age of 63, I loved the parts about having patience and the glass ceiling. My favorite thought: "Recovery is a performance enhancer."

Amelia Vrabel on Patience

"You need to start where you're at. Trust the process and realize that your goals need to be long-term. You can't improve significantly in the short-term, and if you can't keep it up, you won't improve. The bottom line is you'll get better at running if you can do more running. If you're always hurt, you can't do more running."

Amelia Vrabel has been running since 1996, when she started in college to stay fit. Based in Colorado Springs, she completed a 3:26 marathon in Chicago in 2009 and ran her first marathon alongside her mom. Once one of the least athletic kids in high school, Amelia qualified for the Boston Marathon at age 23. She now coaches in the Personal Best Program. She focuses on helping runners develop patience, resilience and a sustainable approach that balances performance with enjoyment of the process.

Connect:
strava.com/athletes/6278182

Full Episode:
extramilest.com/76

The Patient Path to Progress

Many runners want quick results. How do you help them develop a more sustainable mindset?

People always ask me, "When am I going to improve? When am I going to see results?" It's kind of like asking, "When is the tree outside your front yard going to get larger?" You have to plant the seeds, water them and get the sun right, but you don't know what roots are growing underneath that you can't see. It's going to grow when it's ready. Similarly, with your running, you're going to progress based on the conditions you set up. That's why I always tell people to find the wins when they can and celebrate them. You're making progress even when you can't see it. But when you can, that's great.

Get out of your own head. Many people struggle with trying to do what everyone else is doing and feeling like they need to be at a certain pace. When I was little, I thought that if you couldn't run a 10K in 40 minutes, you had no business running. That's humorous now because I know very few people who are faster than that. There's too much focus on training paces and where you should be for this or that. There's a lot of thought that you have to train every day just like you'd race. But no other sport practices that way, so why would running be any different?

What's your approach to long-term running success?

I always tell people, "I'm planning to run when I'm 80." If I thought short-term, I wouldn't be there. Running adds so much to my life when it's a de-stressor, not a stressor. When it becomes a stressor, nobody has time for that because we have other things to accomplish.

It's not how much you train but how much you can absorb. If you simply aren't in the right place to absorb that training, then the training is not really going to help you.

I think people are sometimes afraid because they might have had past experiences where speed work was a suffer fest. It's key to remember that speed work isn't supposed to be painful. Yes, you're supposed to get out of your comfort zone, breathe a little harder and do a little more. But if you're doing it right, you should feel in control. You might be out of your comfort zone, but that's good for you.

Favorite Takeaways from Our YouTube Community

@corwynwarwaruk6807 – Relax more to run faster … so true! When I just relax it's a lot easier to run, easier on my body & just feels better!

@burillakcsaba – No pain, just gain, I would say. Long-term thinking is really important because everything starts with the mental things. Thanks for sharing your thoughts, Amelia, and thanks, Floris, for organizing this interview!

@dirtridergrandpa5873 – For me running at a low heart rate makes it more enjoyable and allows me to run longer distances without pain and long-lasting fatigue. I expect both my time and distance to improve. Thanks for all your podcasts. It has really helped me out as a newer 60-year-old runner!

Scott Frye on Recovery and Mobility

"Give yourself a lot of grace. Don't expect success to come immediately. It's going to take time. It's going to take patience on your part. It is so worth it. I tell you what, once you get on the other side of that mental struggle, it opens up a whole new world, and you just want to keep exploring it."

Scott Frye is a board-certified athletic trainer from Oklahoma City with over 30 years of expertise in injury prevention, rehabilitation and functional training. After 15 years of recreational running, Scott took his training to a new level, setting a marathon personal best of 3:17 on his home course in 2023 and qualifying for the Boston Marathon. With multiple certifications, he's passionate about helping others in their running journeys. Married to wife, Shannon, for 34 years, with two children, Scott lives by the mantra, "You don't have to be great to start, but you have to start to be great."

Connect:
strava.com/athletes/89685446

Full Episode:
Extramilest.com/82

Creating a Body That Thrives

What advice would you give to runners looking to become stronger, healthier and happier in their training and their everyday lives?

When you create an environment in your body that allows it to take care of itself, you'll have a healthier life. The four takeaways are intermittent fasting, cold exposure, proper sleep and caloric restriction.

The body is amazing. It responds well to discomfort and thrives more in discomfort than in comfort. We need to change our mindset from striving for comfort to embracing discomfort. Intermittent fasting lets the body adapt. Cold exposure, whether through cold weather running, cold plunges or cold showers, releases certain enzymes that help the body. Proper sleep is crucial for healing and reducing aging. Caloric restriction doesn't mean starving yourself but being mindful of portion sizes and not always feeling full. These practices help the body thrive better.

How do you stay motivated through the challenges of training?

When you go through the hard times, the rewards and benefits you experience feel so much greater. It's worth it to push through because the feeling of getting to the other side of those struggles is incredibly rewarding.

Get in the habit of daily mobility and strength work; even a few minutes when you're doing the dishes or at a standing desk can make a big difference. The little habits add up and make a long-term impact.

Once you've been through injury and then experience the joy of injury-free running, you find that just moving and being consistent feels fulfilling on its own. The joy of being out there and injury-free keeps you going, and it's a wonderful feeling.

Favorite Takeaways from Our YouTube Community

@rileeb848 – I'm a 38-year-old mom of three with a full-time job. A few months ago, I decided to quit using these blessings (my children and job) as an excuse. I made the choice to start running again. And now I have the opportunity to run every day! The Boston Marathon or NYC Marathon is on my five-year plan. Thank you for keeping me motivated.

@shag377 – My favorite takeaway is what I have seen—go slowly, and be patient. I ran my second 5K in just over 55 minutes. I came in 38 of 38 of the pack and first out of first against the only person who matters.

@benrusher581 – I think the big-picture approach you guys have in this video helps me to relax for my first half-marathon this weekend. Being flexible when I'm feeling the stress levels rise helps me too.

Charlie Engle on Overcoming Adversity

"We get fixated on finishing things when what we need to do is focus entirely on what we're doing right now."

Charlie Engle is a world-renowned ultra-endurance athlete, writer and recovering addict, best known for his extraordinary journey of running across the Sahara Desert and his inspiring story of personal redemption. After battling addiction and overcoming a federal prison sentence, Charlie has transformed his life through the power of running, finding resilience, purpose and freedom in every step. His memoir, *Running Man*, chronicles his experiences of tackling seemingly impossible challenges, from running across vast deserts to maintaining sobriety. With a deep love for adventure and a commitment to pushing his physical and mental limits, Charlie continues to inspire others through his writing, speaking and relentless pursuit of new goals.

Connect:
charlieengle.com

Full Episode:
extramilest.com/1

Pushing Beyond the Breaking Point

You ran across the Sahara Desert, which was 4,500 miles (7,242 km), in 111 days in extreme temperatures. Two marathons a day. How in the world did you do it? What were those first few days like once you started the run?

The first few days were a slow descent into hell. By day seven, it felt like the abyss. My partners, Ray and Kevin, were sick, and the ground temps were 130–135 Fahrenheit (54–57 Celsius). After just one week, we were already three days behind schedule. Everyone was falling apart. But on day eight, I had this realization that I had to approach the run like sobriety, one day at a time. I focused on running a marathon before lunch, taking a nap, and then running another marathon after lunch. I stopped thinking about the finish line and just focused on the next step.

Every 100-miler (161 km) I've done, at some point, I've wanted to quit. But that's what I love. I want to find that point where I can't take it anymore and then keep going. It translates to anyone running their first marathon, half or ultra. Focus on the small goals, and the big goal will come.

You've been through so many highs and lows, from addiction to running across deserts to going to prison. How do you keep coming out stronger?

I think it's about perspective. Life throws bad things at you, fair or unfair, but it's how you react that matters. Bitterness and anger only hurt the person holding on to them. I've learned not to waste energy being angry about things I can't change. Prison was one of those situations where I decided to make the best of it. I read a lot and started writing my book. I ran in place in my cell, did yoga and eventually got over 50 guys running with me. It was a way to stay sane and to help others. My happiness wasn't dependent on the situation. It was up to me.

Surviving Each Moment

Speaking of challenges, you also tried for years to break a sub-3-hour marathon. Can you talk about how you finally did it?

I got sober at 29 and started running marathons. I became obsessed with breaking 3 hours. I was running all these races in Honolulu, San Diego, LA, but I kept coming up just short, like 3:01 or 3:02. Finally, I realized I was making myself miserable. I was so fixated on that time that I wasn't enjoying running anymore. Once I let go and started enjoying the process again, I broke 3 hours and then did it in almost every marathon after that. It's funny how that works. Sometimes you need to let go of the goal to actually achieve it. It's that balance between pushing hard and also knowing when to relax and just enjoy the process. Once I stopped grinding so hard for that sub-3, it came, and I kept hitting it after that.

What kind of mental approach do you use to keep going when things get really tough?

One of the mantras I use is "no big deal." It's actually a phrase I borrowed from my wife, who's survived lymphoma (a cancer of the lymphatic system) three times. She had it once as a child, again as a teenager, and a third time in her twenties. During all those years of chemo, radiation and pain, her mantra was "no big deal." It helped her get through each day, not thinking about the entire disease, but just focusing on surviving each moment. That really puts everything I do into perspective because, for me, running is voluntary. I remind myself that I'm doing this for fun, and if it gets tough, it's still my choice to be there. It helps me push through when things feel impossible.

"No big deal" reminds me to put everything into perspective. It's just running. No one's forcing me to be there. This is what I've chosen to do, so I embrace the suffering. When I hit that wall, I remind myself that I've been through worse, and I can get through this too.

Favorite Takeaways from Our YouTube Community

@akashjalan4663 – This is by far one of the best podcasts of Extramilest, and my two takeaways: 1. No Big Deal—Nothing is big or small/good or bad as long as you are positive or have a positive mindset. 2. Break the miles in small goals in a race and it will be much easier, and enjoyable …

@ChristopherDunn-v4m – Enjoy the process, enjoy the journey.

@pramodsalemaker5393 – Hi Floris, this is an amazing interview and very useful. What I specifically liked was his use of the word SOBRIETY—a couple of times, and I was stuck with that word; however, as the interview unfolded and Charlie kept sharing his life and adventures, it was so clear that Mr. Charlie is a living example of sobriety. His life is inspirational; the 111-days' run, the disciplined life in prison, the community service H2O project. Wow, all that.

Tim Rowberry on Sustainable Training

"A lot of the time everyone has a bias in training. There's something you're going to be too focused on, whether you're an amateur athlete or elite athlete or elite coach. There's always going to be something that you need to back off of like you're focusing too much on. If you're getting bored, it's because you're probably only thinking about one thing."

Tim Rowberry, a coach, former 400 m runner and adventure-driven strategist behind Sifan Hassan's incredible success, shares his unconventional journey from pacing workouts in jeans to coaching at the highest level. Balancing his own running with an athlete's career across middle distances and marathons, Tim embraces creativity and curiosity in training. From early morning runs in Kenya to spontaneous workouts in undershirts, he prioritizes athletes' health, flexibility in goals and lifelong learning. With a focus on building both resilience and joy, Tim brings a fresh approach to elite coaching, proving that with the right mindset, chaos can fuel greatness.

Connect:
instagram.com/rowberry

Full Episode:
extramilest.com/99

Embrace Your Uncertainty

What advice do you have for runners who experience race nerves and self-doubt?

You have to jump in at some point, because you can't fix what you don't know. You have to see what the problems are before you can fix them. And sometimes things just go well.

I think, before we do a lot of these crazy races, we already accept that we might have blown our chances. That's something that we try to come to terms with first. You have to accept what could happen, bad or good, and then be excited that you can see what you just did, and see the results of how that translated to your race.

There's no better way of learning, and there's no better way of figuring out what to do next. That's why running is so addicting. There's always something else.

You should go out of your comfort zone, especially in training. I know so many people who don't ever change what they do. This is the call to you: Change what you're doing. Keep things interesting.

What are some common mistakes that you see runners make, both for elite and recreational runners?

Everyone has a bias in training. Step back as much as you can. Be more balanced in trying to do a little bit of everything instead of trying to be perfect at everything, or perfect at one thing. If you're just trying to balance things out, you're usually going to be better than if you go too far down one road. That's where injuries happen: doing too much of one thing.

Learn what else you can do and learn what you don't know. Try to educate yourself about what other people are doing, and don't be afraid to try what they're doing.

Figure out what makes you interested in running, whether it's exploring or listening to something. There are so many things you can do to make what would normally be boring better.

What closing advice would you share with recreational athletes looking to become stronger, healthier and happier runners?

Most problems start with the feet. Try to do stability stuff, like standing on one foot and other balancing exercises. You need really strong feet.

Grass and barefoot running can be really good in moderation. Strengthen your core and make sure you're getting enough protein. Get your fueling right. You should be eating foods that specifically give you the fuel to recover and prepare for the next workout.

The hard part is just doing little things that make it easier for you to make a schedule. Create habits if you can, even if you just set out running clothes the night before a morning run. It makes a world of difference to be able to just wake up, put on your running clothes, and get out the door. That's half the battle.

Favorite Takeaways from Our YouTube Community

@Aurathegr8t – What stood out for me is when Tim mentioned about running on soft ground about 95% and also taking care of feet.

@brickmarlin557 – There are so many great things in this video! Keeping your training fun and interesting and not burning out. I struggle with the same thing. Also, I love the subject about exploring and getting lost in Kenya. I am a trail runner at heart and love the off-road running!

@connordickey5177 – Great video! I really appreciated what he said about continuing to find ways to make the training enjoyable.

Believe in the Run on Running Gear

"Running shoes are personal. What works for one runner might not work for another. That's why we always say, 'Find what feels good on your feet and makes you excited to go run.'"

Thomas Neuberger, Meaghan Murray and Robbe Reddinger, the team behind Believe in the Run, are among the most trusted voices in running gear reviews. They are as legit and real as it gets. They have tested thousands of running shoes, apparel, hydration systems and accessories to provide unfiltered, practical advice that helps everyday athletes navigate an overwhelming gear market. With different preferences and perspectives, their reviews help runners make informed decisions about what will actually improve their experience.

Connect:
believeintherun.com

Full Episode:
extramilest.com/102

Find the Gear That Works for You

How should runners narrow down the overwhelming number of shoe options available today?

Thomas: There are so many categories now. You've got to start trying shoes. Begin with a basic neutral trainer: simple foam, a good upper. Then you'll figure out whether you prefer something plated for propulsion, or a max-cushioned cruiser, or a rocker bottom.

It's like collecting whiskey. You try one, find your flavor, and then someone recommends another they think you'll love. It gets nuanced. You have to start with a staple, and then you start to figure out what it is that you like about a shoe.

Meaghan: It's pretty overwhelming, especially as a beginner runner to come in and know nothing about shoes.

Robbe: For someone running 20 miles (32 km) a week, a solid daily trainer can do most of the work. Once you're training more seriously, that's where rotation gets fun. You've got your daily trainer for easy miles, a speed shoe for workouts, and a max-cush shoe for recovery days. That's the sweet spot.

Can you break down the different types of running shoes?

Meaghan: There are road-running shoes, there's trail-running shoes, and then once you get into those sectors, there are daily trainers, race day shoes, tempo shoes and recovery shoes.

Robbe: The craziest thing now, especially on the trail side, is you're getting into some really granular stuff like the gravel shoes and terrain-specific shoes. It's insane, but it's super interesting.

Thomas: Every brand has a basic trainer that you start off with. I think that they sit down with their team and they're like, "This is our staple offering." And from there, it kind of goes off in different directions, whether it's adding plates, stack height, softness, whatever.

What's your take on carbon-plated shoes for recreational runners?

Thomas: Totally depends on the runner. Sometimes the carbon plate is there for propulsion. Sometimes it just stiffens soft foam. It can shift load to your Achilles, so it's not for everyone.

Meaghan: I love carbon-plated shoes. I'd run in them every day if I didn't have to test other stuff. That's why brands have started making these "super trainers": daily trainers with great foam and carbon plates, but with more structure so you can use them regularly. If you love how they feel and you're not getting injured, go for it.

Robbe: Yeah. Run in whatever works, as long as you're not getting hurt. I rotate shoes constantly for testing, with different drops and stack heights. I haven't had a major injury in years. If your legs feel good, that's what matters.

As long as you're not getting injured, then do what feels good. Especially since we've learned that carbon-plated shoes offer you that all-around tool where you can go fast and do workouts and do long mileage, but it saves your legs for the next workout or the next day.

What Looks Good Isn't Always Best

What's the #1 mistake runners make when picking shoes?

Thomas: Buying based on looks or trends. I went through the minimal phase. I ended up breaking a bone in my foot just from overuse without having any kind of cushion. I hate the wide-toe-box shoes. They didn't fit me right. Cushion feels great. That's why shoes keep getting taller. It helps you absorb impact and train longer. Barefoot-style shoes just beat up your body if you're doing real mileage.

Meaghan: I'll say the biggest mistake I think new runners make is they buy the shoe size that they wear for casual shoes in running shoes. If you don't go up when your foot expands, obviously you're going to get bloody toenails, blisters, all that stuff.

Robbe: Going cheap on running shoes. People end up in lifestyle shoes, and you see people running in lifestyle shoes. If you go to running shoes on Nike's website or Adidas, they'll show every athletic shoe that they have, pretty much, and it is impossible to discern. You could get the Pegasus on sale for $80, and it'll be almost the same price; and it's a totally different experience.

Any underrated gear that's made a big difference in your running?

Robbe: Merino wool is a life-saver. I love my Smartwool gloves and neck gaiter. It keeps me warm, doesn't stink, and you can wear it in a bunch of ways. A good base layer changes everything in cold weather.

Thomas: People will spend $200–$300 on shoes and then run in cotton socks. Don't do that. Get good socks. It makes a huge difference.

Meaghan: Sports bras with pockets, especially the back pocket for your phone. It's so nice not to carry extra belts or gear. Now they've got like multiple pockets. So, you don't have to carry a belt or anything extra on you.

Avoid Comparisons and Focus on Joy

Have you had any breakthrough moments in your own training or racing?

Meaghan: A few years ago I changed my fueling and hydration strategy. I realized I'd been underfueling on long runs. Once I started taking in enough carbs and electrolytes, I was able to run 20- to 22-milers (32–35 km) at marathon pace and still feel great afterward. I had a six-minute PR in Boston that year and felt the best I ever had in a race.

I literally stopped my watch at the end, and I was like, "Oh man, I must have paused my watch somewhere in the middle of the race because there's no way I just ran a 2:48." Like, absolutely not.

Robbe: Heart rate training helped a lot. My easy runs used to be too fast. Now, even if I'm running a 9:30 min/mile pace (5:54 min/km) in training for a 7:40 min/mile marathon pace (4:46 min/km), I trust the process. I've avoided injury by slowing down and staying consistent.

When I did the heart rate training, it broke me of the Strava mindset because I was running so slow. I was like, I just have to, like, not care what other people see on Strava or think. It's been so much better.

Thomas: My breakthrough was adding speed work. I ran my first three marathons just doing mileage and plateaued. When I started working with a coach and added tempo runs and intervals, I went from 3:59 to 3:20. That got me my Boston Qualifier (BQ). It was a massive shift.

I kept thinking that I would just get faster doing the same thing every day. Like, if I ran 6 miles (10 km) every day and then a long run on the weekend, I would just get faster. And all it did was keep me consistently at one pace.

Any advice for runners who want to become stronger, healthier and happier athletes?

Thomas: Focus on enjoyment. Stop comparing yourself to others, especially runners with similar abilities. That comparison game ruins the joy. Some of my best runs are when I don't care about pace—just being outside, moving and feeling good.

Meaghan: The biggest key is consistency. You can't rely on flashy workouts. The real growth comes from stacking those boring, easy miles day after day. That's what leads to breakthroughs.

Favorite Takeaways From Our YouTube Community:

@soSEW-COB – "I am a sixty-four-year-old runner. My takeaway from this video is that good advice about the right gear can change your running experience and help you get the most out of your running."

@Stewart-px8ow – I never heard of carbon plate shoes until I heard this. After listening to this, I aim to get it.

@andrewromanelli8714 – I really liked Thomas's advice to stop comparing yourself to others. When I start looking at other runners in my age group, it definitely takes away the joy of running for me. Just focus on improving yourself and don't worry about what others are posting!

PART 5

The Journey of the Everyday Athlete

Progress in running isn't always linear. Some of the biggest breakthroughs come from moments when things fall apart.

In this section, I'll share what I've learned from my own failures, from running the World Marathon Majors and from coaching thousands of everyday athletes. These aren't just running lessons, they're life lessons.

You'll discover why failure can be your best teacher if you're willing to listen. No runner, elite or beginner, avoids setbacks completely. The difference is in how you respond. Do you quit? Or do you get curious about what went wrong?

15
Play the Long Game

In our instant-results culture, everyone's chasing the overnight success story. The 30-day transformation. The quick fix. But after years of coaching runners and building my own projects, I've learned a powerful truth: Sustainable progress follows a different timeline.

Compound Improvements

What's transformed my running journey isn't some revolutionary training method; it's embracing small, consistent improvements. These tiny gains compound over time, often invisibly at first, until suddenly you've completely transformed.

Look at my YouTube channel. I don't push out content daily or even weekly. Just one quality episode per month. That's what worked for me. My identity isn't "content creator" but rather to share valuable running and health insights consistently. After ten years of this approach, one video at a time, we've built a community of over 100,000 subscribers.

Systems over Goals

Apply this same thinking to your running. Instead of focusing only on race goals, build running systems that support long-term progress:

- Add no more than 10% weekly training volume (a small, manageable improvement)

- Keep 80% of runs at easy, conversational pace (making the habit sustainable)
- Schedule regular recovery weeks (preventing the habit from breaking down)

The best performers aren't those with the most ambitious goals; they're the ones with the most effective systems. Their success comes from the identity of being someone who trains sustainably, not someone who crushes every workout.

Habit Stacking

As a busy parent working full time, I've had to be strategic with my time. This book was written through habit stacking, attaching 30- to 45-minute writing sessions to my early morning routine before the kids wake up, rather than waiting for perfect writing conditions or marathon sessions.

The Two-Minute Rule

For your health and fitness, focus on making habits easy to start:

- Ten minutes of strength training is better than a theoretical hour-long session
- A lunchtime walk beats waiting for the "perfect" workout window
- Small, consistent nutrition choices outperform periodic diet overhauls

If something feels too hard to start, you haven't broken it down into small enough pieces yet.

> **REMEMBER:** Behaviors followed by immediate rewards get repeated, but the outcomes that matter most come from delayed gratification. A single healthy meal won't visibly change your body. One morning run won't noticeably improve your fitness. But these actions, repeated with devotion over months and years? That's where the ordinary becomes the extraordinary.

Three Foundations for Long Term Running and Health

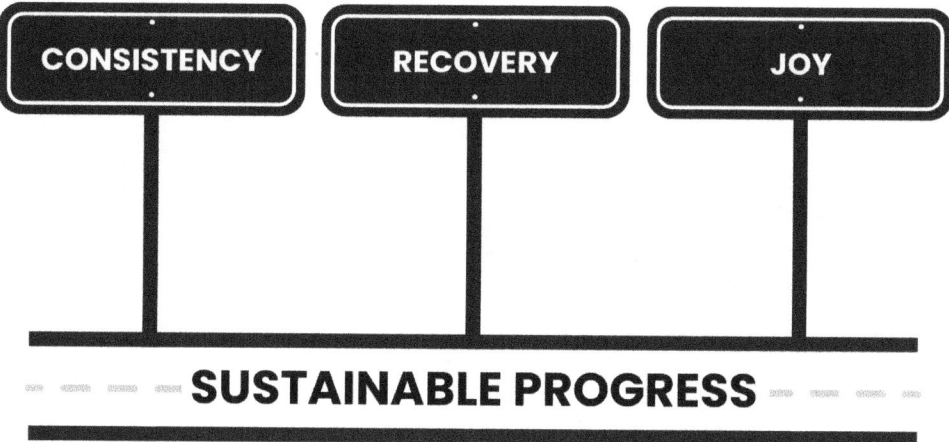

Make It Obvious, Make It Attractive, Make It Easy, Make It Satisfying

The long game isn't glamorous. It won't capture attention at social gatherings or generate immediate validation. It operates quietly, beneath the surface, like roots extending deeper into soil.

But this patience, this willingness to trust the unfolding process, is what ultimately bears the most magnificent fruit. Small actions, repeated faithfully, create a resonance that eventually changes everything.

Chapter Summary

- Sustainable progress follows compound principles. Small, consistent actions repeated over months and years create extraordinary results.
- Build systems and habits rather than just chasing goals. Focus on becoming someone who trains consistently rather than hitting specific times.
- Be patient with plateaus and setbacks, trusting that the process works even when immediate results aren't visible.

16
Dream Big and Visualize Success

Your running journey is as much mental as physical. Visualization and self-belief are powerful tools that can help you achieve what once seemed impossible.

The Power of Visualization

Visualization means creating a detailed mental image of an experience before it happens. This technique engages the same neural pathways activated during physical running, effectively "training" yourself for success. Elite marathoner Eliud Kipchoge famously used visualization to help break the 2-hour marathon barrier.

To implement visualization effectively:

- Find a quiet space where you won't be disturbed
- Create a detailed picture including all senses—what you hear, see, smell, taste and feel
- Focus on key moments like the start, halfway point and final stretch
- Rehearse potential challenges and see yourself overcoming them
- Practice regularly, especially in the weeks before race day

The Belief-Action-Results Cycle

Belief is the foundation of success. When you truly believe in your ability to reach a goal, your actions align with that belief, making success more likely. It follows a powerful cycle:

Beliefs → Actions → Results → Feedback

What separates those who achieve their goals from those who don't isn't just potential but the ability to act on it. Your belief propels you to turn potential into reality, even when the path becomes difficult.

The Vision Board

I use vision boards frequently. A few years ago when I was uncertain about continuing the *Extramilest* podcast, I created a vision board with two bucket-list podcast guests: Eliud Kipchoge and Kilian Jornet. Within only a few months, the teams of both athletes reached out to me to set up interviews. This really opened my eyes to the power of visualization.

To create your own:

- Gather images and inspiring quotes related to your goals in any area of life
- Arrange them visually where you'll see them daily
- Let them reinforce your commitment every time you look at them

Overcoming Doubt

Even with visualization and belief, doubt can emerge during challenging training days. Recognize that doubt is natural but doesn't have to dictate your actions.

"Thought stopping" is an effective technique: consciously interrupting negative thoughts and replacing them with positive affirmations or visualizations of success.

Wim Hof, "The Iceman," shared on *The Extramilest Show* #9:

"The body is capable of amazing things when the mind is clear and focused. Doubt is just an obstacle in the mind, and once you clear it, you open the door to unlimited possibilities."

I've seen it over and over again. Once a runner removes their glass ceiling of limited belief, they can achieve so much more than they initially thought was possible.

Achieving your running goals is as much about the mind as the miles. Dream big, believe in yourself, and visualize your success every step of the way.

Chapter Summary

- Visualization engages the same neural pathways as physical running, effectively "training" your mind and body for success before race day.
- Set bold goals beyond your comfort zone, then break them into daily actionable steps to make dreams reality.
- Use vision boards and mental rehearsal to create daily reinforcement of your commitment and maintain motivation through difficult periods.

17

The Power of Failure in Running and in Life

Let's discuss something most people try to avoid but established athletes learn to embrace: failure.

Playing It Safe Won't Get You Far

Think about your training. If you always stick to the same pace, same routes and same workouts, you might avoid setbacks, but you'll also avoid growth. There's no challenge, no adaptation, no transformation.

The real breakthroughs happen when you take a leap into the unknown, when you push beyond what feels safe. That's where progress lives. Failure isn't something to fear; it's part of the process.

Lessons from My Own Failures

1. The 20-Mile (32-km) Cookie Disaster

One evening, after a long, stressful workday, I set out for a 20-mile (32-km) run commute back home. I didn't take it seriously. I barely ate beforehand and grabbed a pack of vending machine cookies as my only fuel.

The first 15 miles (24 km) were tough but manageable. But when I tried to pick up the pace for the final 5 miles (8 km)? Complete disaster. My energy tanked at mile 17 (27 km). My heart rate spiked. My legs felt like concrete. The last few miles turned into a slow shuffle home.

What did I learn?

- Respect the distance. Long runs aren't something where you can wing it. It's good to stay humble.
- Fueling matters. Cookies don't cut it for endurance, at least not for long runs with race pace.
- It's better to fail in training than on race day.

2. The CIM Marathon Wake-Up Call

At the California International Marathon (CIM), I made another classic mistake. My training had gone well, and I'd originally planned to race by heart rate and feel, focusing on enjoying the experience.

But as race day got closer, some people kept asking: "What's your goal time?" Last minute, I abandoned my initial race plan and went out too aggressively.

What I didn't account for was 90% humidity. By mile 8 (13 km), my heart rate was skyrocketing, breathing became difficult, and I realized it wasn't my day. A few minutes before the finish line I got passed by the sub-3-hour pacers. There was no way I could keep up. I finished in 3:02, far from my PR.

But here's what was most important: I still finished. And after the race, the online running community reminded me that a finish time is just a number. The real victory is pushing through when things don't go according to plan or get tough.

Turning Failure into Fuel

Here's what I've learned: Failure isn't the problem; it's how you respond to it that matters.

When things don't go according to plan:

- Feel the frustration. It's normal.
- Ask yourself, *What can I learn from this?*
- Make adjustments.
- Get back out there. Try again.

And most importantly: Stop caring what other people think. This applies to running, passion projects, work, everything. When you stop worrying about judgment, you free yourself to take risks, fail big and grow even bigger.

Too many athletes obsess over hitting specific times, and they miss the bigger picture. The goal isn't perfection but progress.

If you never fail, you're playing it too safe. The best athletes test their limits, even if it means crashing sometimes. So take that leap. Try something that scares you. And when (not if) you fail, use it as fuel. Because failure isn't the opposite of success; it's a necessary part of it. Keep failing forward!

Case Study — William Barth: Running Full Circle at 70

William Barth had been a runner for over five decades when he joined our PB Program. At nearly 70 years old, his running journey was distinct from many others, filled with early promise, frustrating setbacks and, ultimately, a remarkable renewal.

"In my early teen years, I loved basketball and football. However, in junior high school I discovered track and field. There was something basic and natural about running that attracted me," William explains.

His high school coach taught the Arthur Lydiard "Run to the Top" method, an approach centered on building aerobic endurance through long, slower running, remarkably similar to the heart-rate-based training we emphasize in our program. William was poised to become a standout distance runner, even receiving interest from Dartmouth College, when disaster struck.

"My doctor told me my 'young bones' simply could not tolerate the intensity of my long distance running. My knee cracked open under the stress. Thereafter, my doctor benched me for a whole year, effectively ending any hope I had of running in college."

Despite this crushing setback, William never stopped running. For the next 50+ years, he continued as a recreational runner, always hoping to reach his potential. But he struggled with recurring injuries, torn hamstrings, back problems and cracked vertebrae that kept derailing his progress.

When William discovered our program, he recognized elements of his early Lydiard training but initially resisted the low heart rate approach.

"Having run all my life competitively in marathons, 5Ks, and 10Ks, using this method I just said, it's just too slow. How do you get fast? They say 'run slow to get fast.' That's sort of corny, but there is truth to it."

What kept him committed to the program? "I had no place else to go. I had been injured so badly. If this method doesn't work, what am I going to do? Go out and tear another muscle or break another bone?"

The breakthrough came unexpectedly when William experienced what happens when the approach truly clicks.

"What's really exciting is when you find yourself running at a very fast clip with a low heart rate. That is when the MAF Method really hits home and you go, 'Oh my God, I'm running 9-minute miles (5:36 min/km) and my heart rate is in Zone 2. I'm completely relaxed and yet I'm crushing it.' So imagine what you can do in a race situation!"

William's patience and consistency paid off. He qualified for the Boston Marathon and completed the Chicago Marathon in 3:55, a personal best, despite not fueling optimally during the race. More importantly, he finally found a sustainable way to train without the injuries that had plagued him for decades.

"The PB Program provided me with what was missing in my running journey since my teen years. In short, it filled the void missing in my efforts to make a comeback much later in life. It gives me a vehicle to reach my running potential."

William's advice to runners at any stage is refreshingly straightforward: "Listen to what Floris is talking about. There's a beautiful simplicity to the idea of low heart rate training. The benefits are remarkable: It fights aging, you'll lose weight, and you're going to get fast. That's where the fun part starts, when you find yourself running fast at a low heart rate."

His story shows it's never too late to rewrite your running journey and reach the potential you always knew was there.

Full Episode:
extramilest.com/92

18
Lessons as a Running Coach

Since 2017, I've guided more than 1,000 runners across 60 countries through our PB Program. What follows isn't just advice. It's the distilled wisdom from hundreds of transformations. The patterns I've seen aren't just about running faster but about becoming better versions of ourselves.

Be Kind to Yourself

Most runners I've worked with arrive as their own harshest critics, carrying the weight of expectation heavier than any training load.

Your worth isn't measured in miles or minutes. You are not a collection of splits and statistics. You are the vessel through which the joy of movement flows. When you release the grip of judgment, space opens for transformation.

This isn't just feel-good talk. It's practical! Tension literally restricts your movement. Self-criticism creates physical resistance. Running freely requires letting go of that mental chatter.

Feel, Don't Think

The most profound breakthrough in running happens when you stop watching and start witnessing.

Our culture is data-obsessed with things like heart rate zones, cadence metrics and oxygen uptake. But your body has wisdom that predates technology! It communicates through sensations, rhythm and the conversation between breath and movement.

The runners who make the biggest improvements are those who develop the courage to look beyond their watch data and become more aware of self. They learn to distinguish between productive discomfort and warning signals. They discover their natural cadence, not through counting but through listening.

Your body isn't a computer to program; it's an instrument to play. Learn its music!

The Slow Build

Tiny changes compound into remarkable results over time. That's the magic of consistent training. Chasing immediate results will only set you back.

Your first goal shouldn't be some arbitrary time. It should be enjoying the distance. Feel the rhythm of 5K. Dance with the distance of 10K. Build a relationship with the half-marathon before demanding specific performances.

Speed comes naturally from consistency. You can't force it any more than you can pull a plant to make it grow faster.

Structured Flow

Life rarely follows your training plan! Kids get sick. Work gets crazy. Sleep suffers. The runners who succeed long-term aren't the most disciplined. They're the most adaptable.

Your training schedule should be like water: structured enough to maintain direction, fluid enough to find its way around obstacles.

Listen to what the day is telling you. Some mornings call for intensity; others for gentle movement. Some days demand rest. This responsiveness isn't weakness; it's wisdom.

Slow Down (Seriously!)

There exists an almost universal resistance to slowing down. The ego rebels against ease. Yet paradoxically, deliberate slowness creates the fastest path forward.

When you ease your pace, amazing things happen. Your breathing deepens. Your form improves naturally. Your muscles recruit more efficiently. Your aerobic system strengthens. You build the foundation that later supports those breathtaking speeds.

The best runners I've coached aren't those who push hardest in every workout, but those who embrace the power of ease. They understand that slowness isn't surrender; it's strategy.

Sleep Heals

While you dream, your body rebuilds. Sleep isn't just rest; it's where training adaptations actually happen.

Nobody posts about their eight hours of sleep on Instagram. But those quiet hours in darkness might be the most powerful training you'll ever do.

The runners who improve fastest aren't necessarily those training the hardest. They're the ones recovering most completely. They understand that the work happens on the road, but the transformation happens in bed.

Find Your Community

Running's greatest rewards aren't measured in medals but in connections. The runners who find lasting joy in the sport are those who find their tribe.

We weren't designed to transform alone. When you share your running journey with others, something magical happens. Your challenges resonate. Your victories multiply.

Whether it's joining a local running group, connecting online or just having a few training partners, community matters. It amplifies your commitment, reflects your progress and supports your growth.

Consistency over Perfection

I've seen runners try the most advanced training methods, buy the latest gear and follow complex nutrition plans, yet make little progress. What's missing? Simple consistency.

Be honest with yourself. Are you really showing up regularly?

Your body responds to regular stimulus, not occasional brilliance. Three or four decent runs every week for months will transform you more than sporadic "perfect" workouts.

This is the hidden power of habits: small, consistent actions compounding over time.

The Journey Transforms You

Running isn't just about getting from point A to point B faster. It's about who you become along the way.

Eventually, your fastest mile will slow. Your longest distance may shorten, but the person you become through running—someone who is more resilient and more connected to their body's wisdom—stays with you.

The real finish line isn't marked on any course. It's the moment you realize that running hasn't just changed your body, it has changed your relationship with yourself and the world.

In your footsteps, your breath and the community you build, you discover not just how to run but how to live better every single day.

Chapter Summary

- Practice self-compassion and kindness toward yourself. Self-criticism creates physical tension that restricts movement and limits performance.
- Listen to your body and develop awareness of how you feel, rather than overthinking data. This leads to better training decisions and injury prevention.
- Build community connections for accountability and support while maintaining consistency over perfection in your training approach.

19
World Majors: A Runner's Guide

Few races match the energy of a World Marathon Major. The crowds, the legendary courses, the rush of running through history, it's a race experience unlike any other. After completing the six original World Majors, I've gathered key takeaways that can help you navigate these prestigious races, or any big-city marathon.

1. Arrive Early and Stay Relaxed

World Marathon Majors are massive events with tens of thousands of runners, which means logistics take time. Long bathroom lines, packed starting corrals and bag-drop chaos can throw off your focus if you cut it too close.

Early arrival helps you settle your nerves and get mentally prepared. Nothing creates pre-race anxiety like watching the minutes tick down while you're stuck in a bathroom queue. Give yourself that buffer.

2. Know Your Course; Every Major Has Its Character

Each World Marathon Major has unique challenges:

- **Boston:** Rolling hills throughout, with the infamous Heartbreak Hill at miles 20–21 (32–33 km)
- **New York:** Bridge crossings and elevation changes make pacing tricky

- **Chicago:** Flat and fast, but wind can be a factor, and tall buildings affect GPS
- **Berlin:** The flattest and potentially fastest course, where world records are set
- **Tokyo:** The course includes some sharp turns, but it's relatively flat and fast
- **London:** Relatively flat with a few subtle elevation changes and sharp turns

3. Dial In Your Pacing and Don't Chase the Crowd

The energy at a World Major is electric and intoxicating. It's dangerously easy to get swept up and start too fast.

The most important tip for any of the World Majors is don't start too fast. It's easy to get carried away. This is perhaps the most universal advice for any marathon, but it's especially critical in majors where adrenaline runs higher than usual.

At the 8-mile (13 km) mark in London, I was at 54:20, on pace for a sub-3-hour finish. I felt good but immediately tempered my enthusiasm: "I think it is more of a downhill, with a bit of back wind, so knowing that it's going to get much more challenging, let's focus on one mile at a time."

4. Be Smart About Fueling

One of the biggest mistakes I see runners make at major marathons is underfueling. When you're caught up in the excitement, it's easy to forget your nutrition strategy. Setting an alarm on your GPS watch every 20 or 30 minutes can be a good reminder.

My personal strategy is to take in about 90 grams of carbs per hour. That's three gels of 30 g carbs per hour. Many runners I coach started with consuming only 10–30 grams per hour, which simply isn't enough to maintain energy levels in the later stages of the race.

5. Lean In When It Gets Hard

No matter how well you've trained, marathons get hard. Around miles 20–22 (32–35 km), the real race begins.

At mile 22 (35 km) in London, with just a minute and a half to spare for a sub-3 finish, I reminded myself: "Marathons are hard, and I can do hard things." This mental toolkit is what separates successful marathon experiences from disappointing ones.

6. Don't Experiment on Race Day

Marathon day is not the time to try new shoes, new fuel or an untested pacing strategy.

Training is where you practice everything, from nutrition and hydration to gear and pacing. You don't want to be playing Russian roulette on race day with too many things at stake that might not go according to plan.

7. Crossing the Finish Line Is Always a Win

After crossing the finish line in London and completing my sixth World Major, I was overwhelmed with emotion. In the recap video, I shared: "Even after finishing about 50 marathons, I still get emotional. The feelings were so raw. I had to dig so deep for this race."

Finishing any race, regardless of what time it is, is a huge accomplishment. I'm proud of you for giving it a try, for giving it your best, for getting out there.

Most importantly, enjoy the experience. Don't be overobsessed with time; truly look around you and soak in the marathon race day experience. Moments such as crossing iconic landmarks, high-fiving spectators and seeing the finish line appear in the distance are what you'll remember long after you've forgotten your exact finish time.

florisgierman and **extramilest**
London, England, United Kingdom

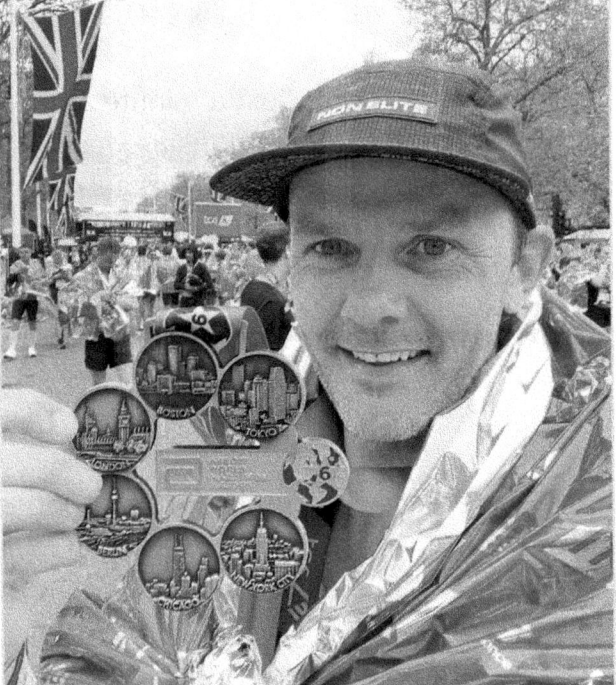

♡ 1,741 💬 277 ⇄ ▽ 50 🔖

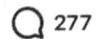 Liked by **pathprojects** and **others**

florisgierman What a beautiful, challenging and rewarding journey this has been. It took me 10 years to complete my 6 Star World Major Marathons.

* Boston in 2:44 (2015)
* New York in 4:38 (2019) pacing my friend Matthew on his first marathon for a @strava project
* Chicago in 2:52 (2022)
* Berlin in 2:57 (2023)
* Tokyo in 2:58 (2024)
* London in 2:58 (2024)

Massive thank you to my wife Jen @zozosadiebug for all your support on this journey. Couldn't have done this without you. Thank you mom, dad and Janneke for inspiring me to try some local 5k's and 10k's growing up. To Sadie and Zoey, this one was for you two, can't wait to show you this beautiful medal soon. Thank you to friends around the world for your support and inspiration.

I'm so happy right now. Much love 😘 🩶

@pathprojects @precisionfandh @corosglobal

#londonmarathon #6star #worldmajormarathon

Case Study — Julianne Dickerson: From Mountain Trails to Marathon Triumph

For Julianne Dickerson from Anchorage, Alaska, running has always been her way to relieve stress and connect with others. Though predominantly a mountain runner, she decided to challenge herself with a road marathon at the California International Marathon.

"When I first switched to running roads, running at the same heart rate I used for trail training felt very difficult," Julianne explains. "It took time to build comfort with running fast on flatter ground."

The PB Program provided what she needed. "I liked having a marathon training program that was time-based and heart-rate-based. It gave me a target for the amount of time I should be spending each day, with quality workouts to build up to the race, while still having flexibility."

The structure and methodology quickly showed results. Julianne's MAF tests showed strong improvement over just three months, from a pace of 7:28 to a 7:05 min/mile (4:38 to 4:24 min/km). "I had 2 miles (3 km) that were 6:59 minutes (4:20 min/km) in my final test. I was really excited because I never had a MAF test with anything that started with a 6."

Her breakthrough workout was a fast-finish long run. "That gave me confidence to start at a reasonable pace in the marathon and finish strong."

On race day, Julianne executed perfectly, starting conservatively and maintaining her heart rate around 171–173 bpm for the first half. Around mile 16 (26 km), we briefly crossed paths.

"You told me to 'Go finish strong,' and I got really motivated," she recalls. "I started running much faster for the next 6 miles (10 km), with several around 6:20 min/mile (3:56 min/km)."

When the inevitable discomfort of the final miles hit, Julianne relied on mental strategies she'd developed: "One thing I try to tell myself is

'Maybe this is what doing well feels like.' You have to try not to judge the effort during the race."

Her disciplined approach paid off spectacularly, and she finished in 2:49:52, 10 minutes faster than her original goal.

"I was very, very happy with the result. Having a detailed written plan helped me be consistent, and it had a very good result. Consistency is very much the key. Having huge volume at low intensity gives you a strong aerobic base that absorbs higher intensity training when needed."

Her parting wisdom: "The question isn't if it's possible, but rather, do you want it? Most people are capable, but you have to know the cost of your goals and be willing to make the necessary sacrifices."

Full Episode:
extramilest.com/29

Chapter Summary

- Study each course's unique challenges (Boston's hills, New York's bridges, Berlin's flatness) and prepare race-specific pacing strategies.
- Prepare thoroughly with logistics planning. Arrive early, know the course, dial in nutrition and manage race day emotions as carefully as physical training.
- Start conservatively despite crowd energy and adrenaline. Disciplined pacing in the first half determines your second-half performance.

PART 6

Recreational Athletes in Conversation

Over the years, as my YouTube channel and podcast grew, I kept hearing requests for more stories from everyday runners. People wanted to hear from others like them: runners balancing work, family and training, figuring out how to improve while juggling everything else in life.

Since 2017, I've coached a lot of these runners through the PB Program, and I've seen just how much progress is possible when you take a smart, sustainable approach to training. Some of these athletes started out injured, overtrained or stuck in a rut. Others just didn't know what to do next. But by making simple changes, they unlocked a whole new level of fitness and enjoyment in their running.

This section dives into stories of real runners, real struggles and real breakthroughs. How did they make it work? What challenges did they face? What advice would they give to others looking to improve? Their journeys show that no matter where you're starting from, there's always room to grow.

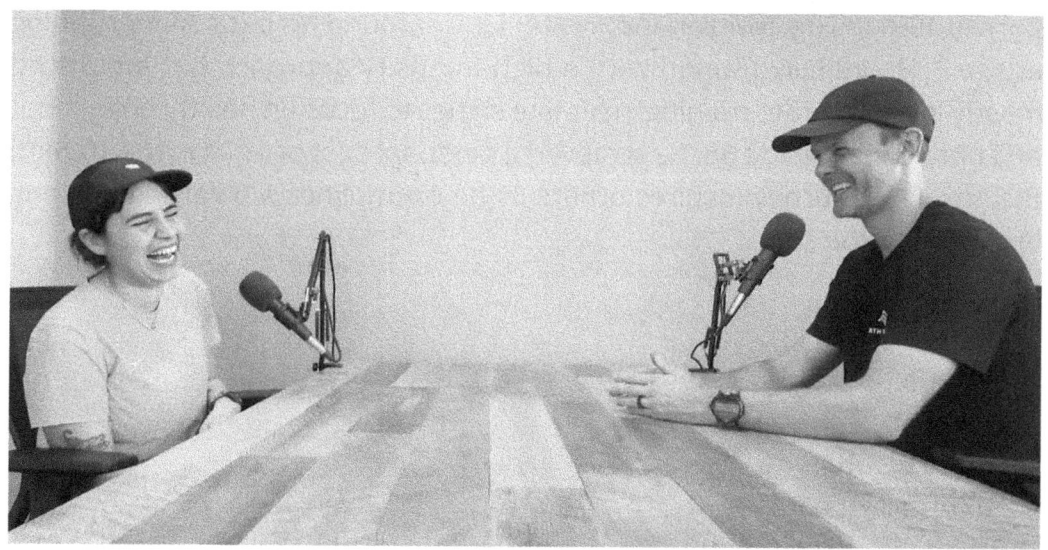

A conversation with Heidi Moreno about finding joy in the journey and experiencing transformation.

Walter Liniger on Joy and Patience

"Be patient and let joy lead your training, not your mind. Who says you have to be fast or strong to be happy? You are living now, not tomorrow or in the next second. This brings a feeling of ease, joy and freedom."

Born in 1951 in Zug, Switzerland, Walter Liniger found his passion for running at age 7. He initially trained with a high-intensity approach but embraced mostly low heart rate training in his late sixties to focus on health, enjoyment and ultra distances. At 68, he achieved a personal best of 11:24 in the 100-km Biel race. His journey inspires others as he exemplifies a balanced, lifelong approach to the sport.

Connect:
strava.com/athletes/14888370

Full Episode:
extramilest.com/44

What advice would you give to runners looking to become stronger, healthier and happier in their training and their everyday lives?

The biggest takeaway for me is the joy of running. Before, I had a love-hate relationship with running. I loved it, but I also dreaded the pain and exhaustion that came with it. Now, with low heart rate training, I enjoy every run. I've also noticed that I haven't had any injuries since I started this approach. It's been a game-changer for me.

You never know what comes around the corner in the next second. You're going to race; you can plan whatever you want, but what will happen will happen as it happens and not in another way. Don't make yourself crazy thinking about how to finish the rest. That will only lead to problems. Stay in the moment where you run, and look at what you've already done, what you already did. That helps.

Kofuzi, a.k.a. Mike Ko, on Training Volume

"People are always asking how to improve their marathon time. The short answer is probably to run more. Slow down your paces, increase your volume and build endurance. If you're getting overuse injuries, you've got to turn down some of those stresses, reduce your intensity, so your body is strong enough to handle it. Then, you can start adding those extra pieces."

Mike Ko, better known as Kofuzi, is a YouTuber and runner from Chicago who has built a strong following by sharing his nonelite running journey and running gear reviews. A father of two, Kofuzi's running story began in middle school, but it wasn't until his thirties, inspired by his dad's marathon goal, that he dove back into the sport after a long hiatus. While his first marathon was a disaster, his dedication to improvement eventually led him to achieve multiple sub-3-hour marathons, a milestone many runners dream of reaching.

Connect:
instagram.com/kofuzi

Full Episode:
extramilest.com/33

Do you have any advice for those looking to improve and become a stronger, healthier and happier athlete?

I think the advice that I generally give to almost every question is to run more. Lately, predominantly, I'm using more of a polarized approach where the vast majority of my running is at my low heart rate range, but a small portion, 10%–20%, is at very, very high intensity. That seems to have really made everything take off.

I've stumbled upon something that really works for me. By running at low intensity, I was able to run consistent 80-mile (129-km) weeks, which was more than I'd ever run. Then on top of that, when I was ready for it, I added some intensity. I was able to add hard work in an 80-mile (129-km) week, and my body is still handling it and able to take it.

For people looking to improve, I think the overall thing would be to run more, but that answer begs another question of "How are you going to run more?" There's a lot more nuance to it. For me, it was to slow down a little bit—build more of a foundation first—and then I could get back to trying to run fast.

John Birtchet-Sharpe on Self-Acceptance

"The most important person that you're running for is the person that you look at in the mirror. Just be honest with yourself and love the journey you're on."

John Birchet-Sharpe, born in 1968, persevered through early health challenges and a near-fatal accident in his twenties before beginning his running journey five years ago. He's made impressive strides, including a personal best of 1:32 in the Manchester Half-Marathon.

Connect:
strava.com/athletes/76038942

Full Episode:
extramilest.com/85

What advice would you give to runners looking to become stronger, healthier and happier in their training and their everyday lives?

Just be happy with yourself. Be happy with the journey you're on. Nobody's looking at you. Nobody really cares about what your Strava time is.

Alcohol is not a friend to running and to health, and I'm not telling anybody not to drink because I've done bloody everything ... but try going out, having a couple of drinks, and then going to bed that night and seeing what it does to your HRV (heart rate variability). It has a big impact, so yeah, alcohol is really not a friend here.

Be kind to yourself in training and don't destroy yourself, but actually go back to getting some of those smaller wins again, like being a little more gentle on the intensity or taking some time off when needed. It's all part of the journey.

Patience is the most important thing. Don't rush to get where you need to get. You will get there. We are capable of more than we think we are. Don't set a roof on your ambitions.

Astrid Feyer Roberts on Injury Prevention

"You have to respect your body and listen to it. If something doesn't feel right, don't push through it. Take it seriously and let yourself recover, or it'll catch up with you."

Astrid Feyer Roberts began running as a child and returned to marathon distances at age 44, after a two-year break. Four years later, she achieved a personal best of 2:47 at the New York Marathon.

Connect:
instagram.com/astrid42.2

Full Episode:
extramilest.com/55

What advice would you give to runners looking to become stronger, healthier and happier in their training and their everyday lives?

There was the saying, like, no pain, no gain, and I took this literally. I learned the hard way that sometimes you have to step back. It's okay to step back when you need it. Sometimes you actually feel that you get a bit tired, or maybe you should rest, and I did not listen to that. I just thought, no, no, the more I train, the harder I train, the faster I will get, and it broke me quite a few times. After my last injury, I had to take six weeks off fully, and that was hard, but I realized patience in recovery is what keeps you strong in the long run.

Todd Marentette on Staying Motivated

"Remember your why, whether it's to lose weight, to feel better or to chase a personal best. Keep that in mind. It'll help you stay motivated when things get tough."

Born in 1977, Todd Marentette took up running in 2016 to lose weight and has since completed 12 marathons, with a personal best of 3:47. He also cohosts *The RUNEGADE Podcast*, where he explores what it truly means to be a runner and a human being.

Connect:
instagram.com/altramarathonman

Full Episode:
extramilest.com/75

What advice would you give to runners looking to become stronger, healthier and happier in their training and their everyday lives?

Don't compare yourself to others because you don't know their whole story. We're all a little bit unique. Progress takes time, and you can't rush it. You want to have a long-term view of it. There's no need to hurry. You have to have that calm confidence that it's okay to take a day off. It's okay to deviate from the plan.

Don't be afraid to ask for help. Find a coach or a mentor who can guide you; someone who's been through it and can offer valuable insights. Do not underestimate the contribution of your feet. Strong feet mean everything.

Eric Floberg on Sub-2:30 Marathons

"Every step is taking you closer to the finish line whether you like it or not. Every day that I work towards this race is another brick stacked forward. When I finally had the humility to actually listen is when I found a huge breakthrough. There's no recipe where people patting you on the back means you'll hit your time goal. Approach each day with the mentality that this is the long game; I'm setting myself up for decades, not just years."

Eric Floberg, a dedicated marathoner, content creator, running coach and father of four from Chicago, shares his journey from a 3:59 marathon to chasing a sub-2:30 finish. He balances high-mileage training with family life and two successful YouTube channels, documenting both his successes and struggles. Eric emphasizes patience, consistency and respecting the marathon distance.

Connect:
instagram.com/eric.floberg

Full Episode:
extramilest.com/96

Do you have any advice for athletes looking to become stronger, healthier and happier runners?

It might sound cliché, but everyone truly is different. Find what works for you and don't stray from it. After eight years, I realized midday running wasn't for me. I needed to wake at 5:00 a.m. for success.

People often start marathoning wanting immediate Boston qualification. You need patience in training but even more patience in discovering what works for you. This comes through trial and error over months and years.

My philosophy is sustainability. Approach each day thinking long-term. You're setting yourself up to run for decades, not just a few years.

My coach Jeff Cunningham taught me about consistency and playing the long game. One of my favorite quotes from him is "You don't always have to have rainbows and glitter shooting out of your ears and butt. Just show up consistently and see what happens."

Jonathan Walton on Success with MAF

"It's a game of patience with Maffetone and low heart rate training. I felt that I wasn't going to get anywhere when I first started. I was probably looking at running 9:30 minutes per mile (5:54 min/km), which for me was ridiculously slow. Then, quite quickly, after about 3 or 4 weeks, the 9:30 min per mile dropped to 9:00 min per mile (5:36 min/km). I kept a record of it and made a graph. I could see the graph going up slightly, and after about 12 weeks, I reached a decent level of fitness."

Jonathan Walton, born in 1969, is a British Masters World Champion marathoner celebrated for his extraordinary progress in long-distance running during his forties and fifties. He achieved a personal best marathon time of 2:28:37 at age 49, and he set the British V55 Marathon record with a stunning 2:32:32 run. Walton attributes some of his success to heart rate training. Initially slowing his pace to adapt, he eventually achieved a MAF pace of 5:55 per mile (3:41 min/km) with a heart rate of 135 bpm. Regularly running over 100 miles (161 kilometers) per week, Walton's disciplined approach has propelled him to elite-level times and inspired countless athletes.

Connect:
strava.com/athletes/8382234

Full Episode:
extramilest.com/15

For people wanting to improve their running, what tips would you share?

I think keeping a record and seeing the gradual improvement was key. Writing everything down, like how I felt during each run, helped me stay motivated. I had different routes: flat, hilly and off-road. I used those to track my improvement.

Patience and consistency are key. Stick with your training, even if you have a dip. Set achievable goals, keep a record of your progress and find what works for you in terms of nutrition and training.

Kathryn Geyer on Finding Joy

"There's so much joy to be had in the movement of your body, whether it's running or something else. We rob ourselves of that joy when it's all about pushing harder."

Kathryn Geyer, born in 1986 in Meredith, New Hampshire, has been running for ten years, regularly completes long distances and has finished her first marathon. Her journey highlights the power of patience and gradual improvement.

Connect:
strava.com/athletes/47096867

Full Episode:
extramilest.com/35

What advice would you give to runners looking to become stronger, healthier and happier in their training and their everyday lives?

If you're finding that on many days of your workout you feel like you want to quit, I'd say question that and experiment with something else. Give it time to evolve, because at first, due to that pressure, it's going to feel like, "I'm not even working out—this is weak; I'm wasting my time." But there's so much joy to be had in this type of exercise and running.

Danny Huibregtse on Enjoyment

"In the beginning, I didn't necessarily enjoy running. I did it to stay fit and to try to stay healthy. But then as soon as I slowed down, it was like, 'Oh wait, I can actually enjoy this.'"

Danny Huibregtse, born in 1990, is a dedicated marathon runner from Westkapelle, the Netherlands. Starting with a marathon time of 3:59, Danny has now lowered his personal best to an impressive 2:29. Danny attributes much of his growth to strategic training and the discovery of low-intensity workouts. A pilot by profession, he's had the unique opportunity to train worldwide, savoring post-run coffee rituals wherever his travels take him.

Connect:
strava.com/athletes/39154584

Full Episode:
extramilest.com/49

What advice would you give to runners looking to become stronger, healthier and happier in their training and their everyday lives?

Your easy runs should be possible breathing through your nose. In my opinion, that's the standard, and if it's difficult, you're running too fast. Sometimes not looking at the watch and running by feel is the best. You could keep your heart rate monitor on and see the data when you get home. But if you go for a run and don't look at the watch, just guess what the values might be. It's a good way to get more understanding of how fit you are at the moment.

Most importantly, make sure you have fun with it. Slow down in the first place. A lot of people don't enjoy running in the beginning because it's too hard on their bodies. They make it too hard for themselves. Slow down, enjoy the run, and don't come home completely wasted. It gives you much more joy, and as soon as you enjoy it, you'll want to do it more. You don't have to force yourself to increase your weekly mileage. It just happens automatically. With that, your speed comes along as well. You'll go faster and faster, and all the benefits come automatically.

Jennifer Kellett on Masters Running

"Our biggest limit is ourselves. Age is not the real barrier that a lot of us think it is. Running isn't just about racing; it's a way of life. I've found so much joy in the journey itself, and I think it's important to embrace that. It's about the day to day, the training and the love of the sport, not just the big events."

Jennifer Kellett, born in May 1955, is an accomplished marathon runner. After beginning to run seriously in 2015 at age 60, Jennifer has set multiple records, including a personal best of 3:23 at the Chicago Marathon, which broke three Australian and world records in her age group.

Connect:
strava.com/athletes/19073319

Full Episode:
extramilest.com/77

What advice would you give to runners looking to become stronger, healthier and happier in their training and their everyday lives?

Consistency is probably the biggest thing, but having said that, flexibility is also important. If you wake up and you don't feel great—if you have had a bad night's sleep—you don't have to stick to that schedule. Your heart and brain don't recognize where the stress is coming from; it just accumulates. You could have stress from family life, work life or physical stress from maybe trying to do too much.

Ben Edusei on Training Fundamentals

"We tend to think we've got to do the full strength or mobility routine; otherwise, it's a waste of time. Make it realistic ... if you can only have two or three minutes a day to do something, use them."

Ben Edusei, born in 1985, is a mobility, strength, conditioning and running coach. With a background in sports science, Ben brings a holistic approach to his coaching and running and has achieved a marathon PB of 3:04. He is especially proud of founding the Zone Blue running group, a community he built to inspire and connect runners.

Connect:
benedusei.com

Full Episodes:
extramilest.com/46
extramilest.com/76

What advice would you give to runners looking to become stronger, healthier and happier in their training and their everyday lives?

Trust the plan, even if you don't see immediate results. Give yourself enough time to build a solid foundation. The fundamentals are key: Focus on base training, mobility and movement work. Look at your stress levels. Consistency is vital, and don't be afraid to fail; it's a learning experience. Something is better than nothing. Even if you're doing something 1% or 2%, that's better than what you were doing a week ago. It's a very slow gradual buildup. Seek advice from others. Don't try to do it all yourself. Surround yourself with mentors, running groups and people who can keep you accountable. I don't even say "failing." It's just been a learning experience. Failing is the best thing for me and has been the most valuable lesson in my life.

Gareth King on Massive Improvement

"A good indicator is if, after a run, you can say to yourself, 'I could do that again.' It's a sign that you're training easy enough."

Gareth King, born in 1980, is an endurance athlete from Northern Ireland who has built an impressive running career by using heart rate training to help transform his marathon time from 3:34 to a personal best of 2:21. With over 20 years of experience, Gareth's proudest moment was representing Great Britain at the 100K World Championships in Berlin, where he finished ninth overall with a time of 6:32:05. He runs for Portadown Running Club and is a devoted husband to Emma and father to their four children.

Connect:
strava.com/athletes/8328371

Full Episode:
extramilest.com/56

What advice would you give to runners looking to become stronger, healthier and happier in their training and their everyday lives?

I think understanding your current fitness level is massive. There's nothing that will tell you that more than running aerobically at a MAF heart rate. If you're down to an 11-minute mile (6:50 min/km), that's where it is. You've really just got to start building from there, and there's no other way around it. If you run way above your current fitness level, it's harder to recover from that. So just really scale it all back and start building from your current fitness level.

Lose the ego; be consistent, and if you're training that way, you should be able to go out every day and build it up gradually. Just be patient; try to clean up the diet, and it will happen. Things will come. Just give it time. As everything develops, you do get stronger and become happier because you're developing and start to embrace it. Everything clicks.

Wissam Kheir on Humility

"Here in Lebanon we have this mentality of 'no pain, no gain.' Well, I didn't know back then that what I was doing was wrong. I was used to the heart rate strap because I liked the biofeedback, but I didn't know how to use the parameters. I thought that hitting 170 heart rate was good. But when I realized that I had to aim for below 135, it was very challenging at first. I couldn't believe that was my fitness level."

Wissam Kheir, born in 1980, is a Lebanese marathon and ultramarathon runner based in Canada. A clinical psychologist and psychotherapist, Wissam is a self-confessed data enthusiast, constantly tracking training metrics and experimenting with new methods, all while discovering Canada's long-distance trails.

Connect:
strava.com/athletes/20155392

Full Episode:
extramilest.com/63

What advice would you give to runners looking to become stronger, healthier and happier in their training and their everyday lives?

Being humble and consistent is key. The benefits of MAF low heart rate training are huge. Coming from a "no pain, no gain" mentality is hard to convert because I saw that here in Lebanon. Other local athletes started using the heart rate concept recently because they saw people like myself adopting this philosophy and seeing benefits, so they shifted.

But the issue was that when they realized this shift required them to slow down, they didn't like the system. So, they said, "No, it's not beneficial. I'm not a fan. This is not for me." As a psychologist, I'm a true believer that MAF has its own people, its own population and its own personalities. You have to let go of your ego and be very humble.

Andy Wheatcroft on Community

"Make running part of your life. If you can build running into your friend network, into how you spend your Saturday morning, into how you travel for work, that you take your running shoes and you find one really cool spot to go running or something, you find it a lot more enjoyable. Enjoy it and find some running friends. They're the best friends on the planet."

Andy Wheatcroft, born in 1967 in Chesterfield, UK, transformed from an "unfit tub of blubber" into a Boston Marathon qualifier through years of dedication. Since taking up running in 2009, he has completed 14 marathons and raised over $125,000 for charity. Now based in Dallas, Texas, Andy is a member of the PB Program and White Rock Running Co-op.

Connect:
strava.com/athletes/48162722

Full Episode:
extramilest.com/89

What advice would you give to runners looking to become stronger, healthier and happier in their training and their everyday lives?

First, take the time to understand your "why." It will evolve, but having a strong reason for running is essential, especially on those tough mornings when motivation is low. My "why" started as running for my kids and for kids in need, but now it's more about being part of a community and running with friends. Second, listen to your body. The most important run is the one that sets you up for tomorrow's run. And finally, set a big, long-term goal, but don't stress about the timeline. Focus on the journey and incremental improvements, and you'll get there.

Josh Sambrook on High Training Volume

"Training at a pace a minute and a half slower per kilometer (2:25 min/per mile) than your race pace just doesn't feel like it makes sense. But using that training technique, it's going to cause the required adaptations. And if you stick with it and trust it, I haven't found anyone who doesn't see really impressive results from doing that."

Josh Sambrook, born in 1996, is a running coach and athlete from Leeds, UK. He is known for his impressive marathon times achieved through a training approach with high volume and minimal speedwork. He ran his first marathon at age 17 and has since completed over a dozen, with a personal best of 2:28.

Connect:
strava.com/athletes/1721750

Full Episodes:
extramilest.com/16
extramilest.com/20

What advice would you give to runners looking to become stronger, healthier and happier in their training and their everyday lives?

I'm a big fan of recording your training. The first thing you've got to do if you want to improve is to keep a record. It almost doesn't matter what you're keeping a record of at the start. But write down what you've done and build from there. Then you can see what's working.

Let's say you do your 5K park run each week. You'll notice yourself getting faster. If you haven't kept a record of what you're doing, it's almost impossible to work out what produced that result. But if you keep a record, you can go, "Okay, well, I ran an extra 10 kilometers this week, and I ran 30 seconds quicker on a 5K."

Keep a record, and then you can work out what works for you and what doesn't. Ditch or change the things that didn't work. That's got to be the secret to continual improvement, using your brain.

Andrea Hudson Baldwin on Visualization

"One thing I do is visualization. Before I ran that Dallas Marathon, I would watch Eliud Kipchoge running there at Monza. I would just absorb his running and his smile and everything. Sometimes I like to visualize Sarah Hall when she's running the end of the race in the rain in London, leaving nothing on the course."

Andrea Hudson Baldwin, born in 1959, is a dedicated runner and family nurse practitioner based in Dallas, Texas. Since starting consistent training in 2015, Andrea has achieved personal records across all race distances, with her marathon PR of 3:28:11 set at the Chicago Marathon. Starting college as a single mom at 45 and graduating at 51, Andrea brings resilience to both her career and running.

Connect:
strava.com/athletes/16598442

Full Episode:
extramilest.com/57

Ash Lewis on His Comeback Story

"I never thought I would run again, but I was inspired by others who found their way back. It showed me that no matter how impossible something seems, you can always come back. Sometimes, it's the small steps that make the biggest difference. You don't have to go from zero to a marathon overnight, but every step you take brings you closer to where you want to be."

Ash Lewis, from Jersey, UK, has an incredibly inspiring story of overcoming challenges. At age 28, he experienced a spinal injury that left him paralyzed from the waist down, and he had to completely relearn how to walk. Today, running has become a powerful driver of momentum in his life. Ash has since run multiple sub-3-hour marathons with a personal best finish of 2:52 at the Manchester Marathon. He is also an accomplished tattoo artist with more than a decade of experience. Ash recently completed a 60K ultramarathon around the island of Jersey.

Connect:
strava.com/athletes/56526119

Full Episode:
extramilest.com/45

Albert Shank on Ultrarunning

"Try not to be too obsessive for too long because that can really kill your running. I've seen it too many times where runners get fixated on maintaining a certain pace or mileage, and then they get broken. Nobody wants to get hurt and not train; that's uncool. So, enjoy what you're doing, have fun, try not to overobsess, and make most of your running very easy. You'll do those hard runs better and get more benefit out of your training."

Albert Shank, born in 1968, is an ultrarunner with fourteen 50K, ten 50-mile (80-km) and one finish at the Mogollon Monster 100. He's been hitting the trails in Phoenix since 1993 and inspiring college students as a Spanish teacher.

Connect:
strava.com/athletes/26803675

Full Episode:
extramilest.com/36

Bill Callahan on Mental Strategies

"I'm a big fan of writing things on my arm. I put someone's name on my arm. It's usually all my family members, and I dedicate every mile to them. I just go, this is for this person, and I start thinking about what that person did for me while I was training for that event. Immediately I start calming down, my heart rate goes down a little bit. It has definitely worked."

Bill Callahan, a runner from central New York state, has lowered his marathon time from 3:40 to 2:50 and completed multiple World Marathon Majors under 3 hours after age 40, inspired by his wife and the memory of his father.

Connect:
strava.com/athletes/14456219

Full Episode:
extramilest.com/13

Larisa Dannis MacFadden on Intuitive Training

"I've made my biggest improvements when I've run for the right reasons and focused on the types of running that excite me most. When you're truly excited about your goals, progress comes naturally. I no longer follow a rigid schedule. I gauge the volume I can handle and see if I can increase it gradually. Day to day, I keep it simple and run based on feel."

Larisa Dannis MacFadden, a road and ultrarunner with a marathon PB of 2:44 and a second-place finish at Western States 100, inspires others with her holistic approach to running.

Connect:
strava.com/athletes/1872175

Full Episode:
extramilest.com/23

Nicki Hugie Terry on Body Awareness

"Instead of training for a pace, I just train by listening to my body. Then, when I get about a month out from the race, I start to assess what type of fitness I am in, and that's when I set my goal."

Nicki Hugie Terry, born in 1984, is a dedicated runner, mother and nurse practitioner. She's run five sub-3-hour marathons, set a PR of 2:55, and completed marathons in 31 states, all while balancing life's commitments and enjoying training runs with her kids.

Full Episode:
extramilest.com/2

Calvin Sambrook on Age Barriers

"I hear a lot of people of my age sort of using age, not quite as an excuse, but maybe it's in the back of their mind as something that might hold them back. It really isn't a factor. You can still get the result. Maybe you have to put a few more kilometers in than somebody in their twenties, but you still get the result."

Calvin Sambrook, born in 1963, transformed his marathon performance from needing rescue in his first attempt to achieving a 3:15 personal best at age 56 in the London Marathon through high-volume, low-intensity training.

Connect:
strava.com/athletes/1722521

Full Episode:
extramilest.com/20

Greg Nance on Taking the Leap

"Start before you're ready. You gotta take the leap. None of us were ever really ready. You have to figure out how to train, how to prepare yourself step by step by step, as you go."

Greg Nance, born in 1988, completed the World Marathon Challenge, running seven marathons on seven continents in seven days. He has been running for more than 30 years, including ultra-endurance events and a 3,156-mile (5,079-km) coast-to-coast run across America for youth mental health.

Connect:
instagram.com/gregrunsfar

Full Episode:
extramilest.com/14

Jay Motley on Overcoming Barriers

"Every mile, every hurdle and every victory, even the tough ones, are part of the journey. Embrace each step as a lesson because they're all helping you grow stronger."

Jay Motley, born in 1980, overcame setbacks to achieve a 2:50 marathon PB and Boston Qualifier at the Hawaii Bird Marathon, and now combines his passions for mental health, fitness and lifestyle medicine as the founder of MindWell Health.

Connect:
strava.com/athletes/5329618

Full Episode:
extramilest.com/11

Kyle Whalum on Mindful Running

"Running is a practice, so you're never going to perfect it. Try this little tweak, this new system or this way of thinking about your form. To me, that's what running is: a combination of being willing to learn and improve, being a student of the practice and just having fun. That's the whole reason we're doing it in the first place."

Kyle Whalum, born in 1983, is a Los Angeles–based ultrarunner and professional bassist with over 25 ultras completed, including a 23:31 personal best at the Coldwater Rumble 100-miler (161 km); he advocates for greater mental health and neurodiversity awareness while balancing his passions for music, mindfulness and movement.

Connect:
instagram.com/kylewhalum

Full Episode:
extramilest.com/71

Liam Lonsdale on the Benefits of Trail Running

"Trails are such good cross-training, even if you're a road runner. With stability and climbs, you're building up different muscles. It's generally lower impact than running on the road. Just factor in at least one trail session a week, and you will get stronger."

Liam Lonsdale, born in 1989, is a seminomadic trail runner, professional photographer, DJ and father of two, who combines his love for the mountains and adventure with his passion for building running communities in Oakland and Mexico.

Connect:
liamlonsdale.com

Full Episode:
extramilest.com/78

Martinus Evans on Inclusivity

"Comparison is the thief of joy. You have to be consistent and persistent in your own journey. You can't look to the next guy or the next girl beside you. Running has helped me figure that out, to understand that there's no such thing as a failure and no such thing as a loss. All of this is a learning instrument to keep us going through our life."

Martinus Evans, founder of the Slow AF Run Club, is an inspiring marathoner, coach and advocate for inclusivity in running. With over a decade of experience and eight marathons completed, he is dedicated to creating spaces where every pace and body type is celebrated.

Connect:
300poundsandrunning.com

Full Episode:
extramilest.com/65

Michael Ovens on Morning Runs

"I urge everyone to set their alarm for an hour before they normally get up and just give early morning runs a go. It's a really good start to your day."

Michael Ovens, born in 1978, is a runner from Jersey in the UK who improved his marathon time from 5:11 to 3:18, completing three 48-mile (77-km) ultras and crediting his success to a focused training plan, quitting alcohol and prioritizing recovery.

Connect:
strava.com/athletes/12746394

Full Episode:
extramilest.com/19

Jessica Dorsey on Mental Strength

"Even when it gets dark, sometimes I just need to laugh it off or smile to help get through it."

Jessica Dorsey, a mother and marathoner with a 2:53 PB at Grandma's Marathon, has probably done more pushups and pull-ups than you!

Connect:
instagram.com/mamainthefastlane

Full Episode:
extramilest.com/12

Kelley Puckett on Racing Strategy

"When you're at the end of a marathon and your mind is telling you to stop, try going faster. Because really what you need is just to change your legs. You need some kind of change. Mentally wrap your head around the fact that you're not gonna die if you do. If it backfires, then you pull back."

Kelley Elizabeth Puckett has completed over 30 marathons, including prestigious ultras like Badwater 135 and AC100, achieving a sub-3 marathon at California International Marathon (CIM) while maintaining a balanced approach that combines structured training with joy.

Connect:
linkedin.com/in/kelley-puckett

Full Episode:
extramilest.com/12

Gwen Ostrosky on Breakthroughs

"Still throw in a run that's not about time. Leave your watch at home and just enjoy running."

Gwen Ostrosky transformed from a sprinter to marathoner, breaking through a 3:30 plateau to achieve a sub-3-hour marathon at California International Marathon (CIM) through focused training and community support.

Connect:
instagram.com/princessgwendolyn

Full Episode:
extramilest.com/12

Andy Hooks on the Love of Running

"My mindset changed ... it became a lot less about trying to qualify for Boston but became more of a love of running. That part is what allowed me to become a better runner."

Andy Hooks, born in 1981, is an accomplished runner and ER nurse from San Antonio, Texas, with a marathon PR of 2:45, a 100K win in 9:15 and a passion for health and technology.

Connect:
strava.com/athletes/23698843

Full Episodes:
extramilest.com/21
extramilest.com/37

PART 7
Gear, Resources and Final Insights

Running is a beautifully simple sport. Just lace up and go. But as you progress, the right gear can make a significant difference in your comfort, performance and longevity as a runner. After exploring training methods, elite wisdom and performance science in previous sections, it's time to address the practical elements that can enhance your daily running experience.

In this section, I'll share what I've learned about running equipment after years of personal experience and conversations with experts. From finding the perfect running shoes and using GPS watches effectively, to selecting clothing that prevents chafing and hydration systems that don't disrupt your form, you'll learn what genuinely matters and what's just marketing hype. The right gear won't transform you overnight, but it can make your journey more comfortable and sustainable.

I share my most valuable resources, the podcast episodes runners have found most life-changing, the websites and tools that have helped thousands reach their personal best and guidance on when additional support might accelerate your progress. Running isn't about chasing the latest trends; it's about discovering what genuinely works for your unique body and keeping things beautifully simple.

20
Gear Up — Recommendations for Runners

A list of my favorite running gear and tools, including some discount codes for our Extramilest Community can be found at florisgierman.com/resources.

GPS Watches and Heart Rate Monitors

Watches and heart rate monitors are two valuable tools in any runner's arsenal. Tracking your heart rate helps you train at the right intensity, making sure you're not pushing too hard on easy days or taking it too easy during hard workouts.

I've discovered that not all heart rate monitors give you the same results. Most GPS watches come with built-in optical sensors that measure your pulse from your wrist. While convenient, these sensors tend to be less accurate than a chest strap or armband, especially when you're running on trails or uneven terrain.

My recommendation? Use a separate heart rate chest strap or armband rather than relying solely on your watch's wrist sensor. Brands like Coros, Garmin, Polar and Wahoo provide reliable readings that help you stay in your target zone.

When choosing a GPS watch, focus on the basics first. You don't need the most advanced model with every feature imaginable. Start with a watch that pairs easily with your heart rate monitor and has the option to add a heart rate alarm, if that's something you find helpful. The fancy features might look cool, but most runners end up using just a handful of core functions.

Running Shoes: Finding the Perfect Fit

Shoes are the foundation of your running gear. A well-fitting pair can prevent injury, while poorly fitted shoes can lead to discomfort and long-term problems.

One of the most common mistakes I see new runners make is choosing shoes that are too small. Your feet expand during long runs, and having extra room in the toe box can make all the difference in your comfort and foot health.

Through my work with Lawrence van Lingen, I've learned that modern "Super Shoes" are designed to compress and spring back like a pogo stick, which can actually help improve running form. Lawrence believes Super Shoes encourage a more effective running pattern: "land, load, explode."

Lawrence has pointed out how Super Shoes have led to dramatic improvements in people's running form. In the past, many runners were focused on decreasing ground contact time and avoiding impact, which led to picking feet up too quickly rather than driving forward with confidence. He's also observed that Super Shoes have allowed many runners to handle higher weekly mileage that they couldn't manage before, and have even helped some elderly runners who previously couldn't run at all to get back out there.

From my own experience, I've found that Super Shoes with carbon plates are best viewed as the "icing on the cake." While many runners make these shoes a top priority to shave off time, I believe consistent running, quality sleep, proper stress management and good nutrition are far more important foundations for improvement.

If you decide to try Super Shoes, I recommend easing into them gradually. They can feel significantly different at first. I suggest starting with some shorter runs, then incorporating a few long runs and tempo sessions before racing in them. This approach helps your body adapt to the different mechanics and feel of the shoes.

I've found that wearing the least amount of shoe you can safely run in encourages better form. This approach reduces reliance on excessive cushioning and promotes natural movement. That said, not everyone should jump into minimalist shoes, especially if you're transitioning from traditional running shoes.

Visiting a specialty running store to have your gait analyzed is a great first step. Different runners have different needs. I've noticed some runners prefer more cushioned shoes for longer distances, while others opt for lightweight trainers for speed sessions.

A good rule of thumb is to find the balance between support and flexibility, allowing your foot to move naturally while still providing protection. Whether you prefer the barefoot feel of a Vivo barefoot shoe or the cushion of a HOKA, choose a shoe that complements your running form and environment.

Running Clothing: Comfort Comes First

The right clothes can significantly enhance your performance. Look for moisture-wicking, breathable fabrics that help regulate your body temperature.

One mistake I made for years, especially in cooler weather, was overdressing. I've since learned that when you start your run, it's actually good to feel a little cold. Your body warms up after the first 10–15 minutes, and overdressing leads to overheating, making it harder to keep your heart rate down during long runs.

Chafing is another common issue that can turn an enjoyable run into a painful experience. I've found that using anti-chafe products like Squirrel's Nut Butter or Body Glide works wonders, especially on hot days or during long runs. This small addition to your gear kit can make a massive difference in comfort.

A separate short and base liner from Path Projects, the company I cofounded, can also significantly reduce chances of chafing.

Hydration and Nutrition Gear

Whether you prefer handheld bottles, waist packs or hydration vests, the key is having easy access to water during your runs. For longer races and ultramarathons, I've found that a hydration vest is invaluable. It allows you to carry water, gels and other essentials while distributing the weight evenly across your body.

For shorter runs, a handheld water bottle or a simple waist pack might be sufficient. The goal is to choose a system that doesn't disrupt your running form and keeps you hydrated without weighing you down too much.

Tools for Data-Driven Runners

Power meters, heart rate variability monitors and sleep trackers are becoming more popular for runners interested in diving deep into data. However, I've learned that it's essential to use these tools wisely and remember that what your body tells you is often more important than what a device says.

Tracking your heart rate variability can provide insights into how well your body is recovering, but it's just one piece of the puzzle. Ultimately, running is about listening to your body and not getting too caught up in the numbers. An over-reliance on technology can sometimes take away from the joy of running.

Keep It Simple

The running industry constantly bombards us with new products. Every season brings the latest shoes, watches and gadgets, each claiming to be the revolutionary tool that will transform your running. I've learned to see through the marketing hype.

Here's what I believe after years of running and coaching: The best gear is what works for you and your unique body. It doesn't need to be expensive or trendy. It just needs to support how you naturally move. I've seen runners set personal records in basic shoes while others struggle despite wearing the most advanced technology money can buy.

The reality is that consistency in training, adequate recovery and smart nutrition will improve your running far more than any piece of gear. When I talk with the most successful long-term runners, they rarely credit their success to having the perfect gear. Instead, they point to developing a sustainable running practice and learning to listen to their bodies.

As you navigate the overwhelming world of running gear, keep bringing yourself back to this question: "Does this support my natural movement, or is it trying to compensate for or restrict it?" The best gear enhances your running experience while allowing your body to move as it was designed to do.

So keep it simple. Find what works, stick with it and spend more energy enjoying your runs than worrying about what you're wearing on them.

Case Study — Brent Cunningham's Journey to Boston

"What a difference a year makes," Brent Cunningham shared in our PB Program community. "Change your nutrition, do MAF training and reduce stress in your life, and look what happens!"

The transformation in this 57-year-old Seattle-area runner was nothing short of remarkable. Comparing his Deception Pass 25K trail race results side by side told the story: In just one year, his finish time dropped from 3:31:24 to 2:38:04, improving his pace from 14:28 to 10:43 per mile (8:59 to 6:40 per km). Meanwhile, his weight dropped from 175 to 152 pounds (79 to 69 kg).

From Boston to Burnout and Back

Brent was no stranger to achievement. He had completed the Boston Marathon in 2013, the year of the bombing, and had experienced first-hand the electricity of that iconic race. But life took a turn when a job promotion led to increased stress and declining health habits.

"I gained 30 pounds (13.6 kg) over a five-and-a-half-year period," Brent explains. "I was still moving my body quite a bit, but I turned to food, especially sugar and processed foods, to comfort me during challenging times."

When a fellow trail runner mentioned the low heart rate training, Brent was intrigued but skeptical. His first MAF test was humbling, a 12-minute-mile pace (7:27/km) that felt almost embarrassing.

"There are dogs walking who are going to pass me," he says with a laugh.

The Power of Patience

"Slow progress. I'm getting there," became Brent's mantra as he patiently tracked his improvement through regular MAF tests. The numbers tell the story of how his running pace improved at a heart rate of 123 beats per minute:

**Brent's Running Pace over 12 Months
at a Heart Rate of 123 Beats per Minute**

MONTH	ZONE 2 (MIN/MILE)	ZONE 2 (MIN/KM)
MONTH 1	12:14 MIN / MILE	7:36 MIN / KM
MONTH 2	11:46 MIN / MILE	7:19 MIN / KM
MONTH 3	10:50 MIN / MILE	6:44 MIN / KM
MONTH 6	10:18 MIN / MILE	6:24 MIN / KM
MONTH 7	9:54 MIN / MILE	6:09 MIN / KM
MONTH 8	9:24 MIN / MILE	5:50 MIN / KM
MONTH 10	9:07 MIN / MILE	5:40 MIN / KM
MONTH 12	8:48 MIN / MILE	5:28 MIN / KM

"It just takes consistency over time," Brent reflects.

The real breakthrough came when he overhauled his nutrition, eliminating coffee creamer, sugar and processed foods. Instead, he focused on whole foods, meat, fruit, vegetables and complex carbohydrates. Combined with intermittent fasting and increased water intake, he felt his transformation accelerate.

"I cut way back on sugar and processed foods, eating more fruit and vegetables and drinking more water. The PB Program is a huge WIN!"

A Dream Reborn

Today, Brent's sights are set firmly on a return to Boston. "Dream: for Boston next fall. I'll be in the 60–65 age group. Living the dream!"

With his improved fitness and his new age group, he believes qualifying is within reach. "I'm training for the CIM. My dream would be to qualify for Boston again. I need to run a 3:35 marathon!"

For Brent, the benefits extend far beyond running faster. "It's about becoming strong and awake for love's sake," he shares. "The mental health and emotional health side of all these things is really helping me too.

"Give yourself freedom to dream in different areas of your life. Set a goal and then go slow. You don't have to sprint. Just start making baby steps and go for it."

Full Episode:
extramilest.com/91

Chapter Summary

- Choose gear that supports your natural movement rather than restricting it. Heart rate chest straps provide more accurate readings than wrist sensors.
- Keep it simple and focus on comfort. Breathable clothing, proper shoe fit and anti-chafe solutions matter more than expensive technology.
- Remember that consistency in training, recovery and nutrition will improve your running far more than any piece of gear.

21
If You're Feeling Down, Read This

If you're reading this chapter because everything feels overwhelming right now, I want you to know something important. You're enough just as you are. Sometimes we just need to pause and listen to what our body and heart are telling us. I've sat exactly where you're sitting.

You matter. Your struggles are real. And things can get better.

> **IMPORTANT NOTE:** This chapter shares personal experiences and general wellness strategies. If you're experiencing serious mental health challenges, please reach out to a qualified mental health professional. You deserve support.
>
> **Crisis Resources:**
>
> – U.S.: 988 (Suicide & Crisis Lifeline)
> – International: findahelpline.com

You're Not Alone

Whether you're feeling totally overwhelmed by life, or dealing with anxiety that won't quit or a complete lack of motivation or deep sadness, know that you're not alone in this. I've sat exactly where you're sitting, and so have many runners in our community.

Sometimes life hits us like hitting the wall at mile 20 of a marathon. Everything that seemed manageable suddenly feels impossible. Your mind starts playing tricks on you. That voice in your head telling you to quit gets louder.

If this sounds familiar right now, please know that these feelings are temporary, even when they don't feel that way.

You're Enough

You're not broken or damaged. Sometimes, we just need to pause and listen to what our body and heart are telling us. You're human, and you're dealing with something incredibly difficult that takes real courage, even when it doesn't feel courageous at all.

Right now you might be in the mud, but here's what I know: The most beautiful flowers grow from mud. Your struggles don't define your worth. They're part of your story, but they're not the end of it.

Breaking the Loop

Here's something that might surprise you. About 90% of our thoughts are the same every single day. When we're struggling, those thoughts sound like broken records: "I'm overwhelmed"; "Nothing's working for me"; "I'm not good enough."

These aren't just random thoughts. They're creating your reality. Every time you think a thought, your brain releases chemicals that make your body feel exactly what you're thinking. Think stress, feel stress. But here's the beautiful part. This same process works in reverse.

The moment you become aware of these repetitive thoughts, you've taken the first step toward freedom. You're not your thoughts. You're the observer of your thoughts. And that observer has the power to choose differently.

> **SIMPLE PRACTICE:** When you notice your mind running familiar loops of worry, place your hand about two inches below your navel and breathe into that space for 30 seconds. This isn't about forcing positive thoughts. It's about coming back to the present moment, where your power actually lives.

Movement as Medicine

Daniel Edwards, a runner in our PB Program, shared something powerful. "For me, the mental health benefits of running have been even more important than any physical gains. Running consistently has been essential to my recovery journey."

Daniel's journey began in one of the darkest places. He had attempted suicide and was battling severe depression. Movement became his lifeline back to hope.

What Daniel discovered matches what researchers have proven. Consistent movement can be as effective as medication for treating depression and anxiety. But there's something deeper happening when we move our bodies.

Most of us spend our days lost in thought, replaying past hurts or worrying about the future. When we're not present, our energy goes down. Movement, even gentle movement, brings us back to this moment, interrupting negative thought patterns.

Start Where You Are

Starting doesn't require feeling ready or motivated. It just requires the smallest step forward, whatever that looks like for you today.

- **If running feels impossible:** Walk slowly around your block.
- **If that seems too much:** Step outside for 5 minutes and breathe.
- **If even that feels overwhelming:** Stand by an open window and notice the air on your skin.

Your body has carried you through every difficult day of your life so far. It deserves your kindness, not your criticism.

> **TRY THIS:** For the next three days, move your body for just 5 minutes daily. It could be walking, stretching, dancing to one song or doing jumping jacks. The goal isn't fitness. It's proving to yourself that you can show up.

Keep showing up, even when it's tough. Every athlete faces days when everything feels harder than it should. It's natural to feel frustrated or beaten down sometimes. That doesn't make you weak. It makes you human. Missing the mark is part of the process.

Creating New Stories

Here's something I've learned. We're all creators, not victims. Everything that happens is happening for us, not to us. This isn't about toxic positivity or pretending everything is fine. It's about recognizing your power to respond differently.

To create something different, you have to become someone different. This isn't about changing overnight. It's about small, daily choices to think differently, move differently or be present differently.

> **VISUALIZATION PRACTICE:** Spend 2–3 minutes each day imagining the version of yourself that has moved through this difficult time. How does this future self wake up? How do they treat their body? How do they respond to challenges?
>
> This isn't fantasy. This is you creating a map to your future.

The Compound Effect of Small Steps

Change doesn't always feel good, but when you have a clear vision of where you're headed, you can lean into the discomfort knowing it's temporary.

These small choices compound over time. You might not notice the difference today or tomorrow, but in a few weeks, you'll look back and see how far you've come.

Writing Your Comeback Story

Your story isn't over. This difficult chapter you're in right now? It's not the ending. It's the part where the hero discovers their strength.

Every runner knows that the hardest miles often come right before the breakthrough. The same is true in life. Your willingness to keep moving forward, even when it's hard, is already proof of your resilience.

Next Steps

You don't have to figure everything out today. You just have to take the next small step.

Movement doesn't have to be perfect or impressive. Meditation can be three deep breaths with your hand on your heart. Progress doesn't have to be dramatic to be real.

Give yourself grace. You're doing the best you can with what you have right now, and that's enough.

Every time you choose presence over panic, movement over stagnation, hope over despair, you're literally rewiring your brain for healing.

We're Here with You

Whether you're taking your first steps or you've been moving for years, our community understands that some days the hardest part isn't the physical challenge. It's showing up when your heart feels heavy.

We see you. We believe in you. And we're here to walk, run and move forward alongside you, at whatever pace feels right.

> **REMEMBER:** It's okay to ask for help. Reaching out isn't a sign of weakness. It's a sign of strength. Keep moving forward, even when it's hard. Trust that things can get better.

Show up daily, catch yourself when you default to old patterns and gently bring yourself back to the present moment.

You've got what it takes to get through this. You are the creator of your life, and this moment right now is where your power lives.

Chapter Summary

- You are enough just as you are. The struggles you're facing are temporary, and this difficult chapter isn't the end of your story.
- Start small with gentle movements, like 5-minute walks, to break negative thought cycles and create space for healing.
- Seek support when needed and choose resilience by reframing challenges as opportunities to grow stronger in running and life.

22
Lessons from My First 100 Mile (161 km) Run

At age 32, I set out to do something I had never attempted before: run 100 miles (161 km) from Los Angeles to San Diego. No crew, no pacers, no aid stations; just me, my hydration vest packed with water and snacks, and the open road ahead.

I started at 2 a.m. while the city slept. The only sounds were my footsteps and the occasional passing car. It was the hardest thing I've ever done, physically and mentally.

The first few hours felt surprisingly good. By the marathon mark in Newport Beach (3:40), I noticed my heart rate was higher than planned, an early warning sign I chose to ignore. At Monarch Beach, 35 miles and 5 hours in (56 km), I remember thinking, "Feels like I'm just getting started." Oh, how wrong I was!

Through Camp Pendleton at mile 61 (98 km), reality hit hard; I had severely underestimated this run. By mile 62.6 (100 km), at 9:23 into the run, I hit my lowest point ever in running. I remember talking to myself: "Stay calm. The only thing I can control right now is my attitude and how I respond."

Finally, after 17 hours and 47 minutes, I completed the full 100 miles (161 km) in San Diego.

3 Lessons Learned from Running My First 100-Miler (161 km)

Lesson 1: Pace Yourself (No, Really, Slow Down!)

Look, we've all heard "start slow" before, but 100 miles (161 km) has a way of teaching this lesson like nothing else. I crushed the first 50 miles (80 km) in 7 hours 17 minutes, thinking I could maintain that pace. My legs had other ideas. The second 50 miles (80 km)? A humbling 10 hours and 30 minutes, more than 3 hours slower than the first half.

The lesson? If you start too fast in a long race, the price you pay later is brutal when you are forced to slow down.

Lesson 2: Sugar and Caffeine Can Bring You Back to Life!

Around the 50-mile (80-km) mark, I got sloppy with my nutrition and hydration intake. My energy plummeted, my heart rate spiked, and I hit the wall hard.

Then came the magic. I drank a Coke. Within minutes, it was like someone flipped a switch. The fog lifted, my legs remembered how to run, and I was back in business. I had never experienced such an instant turnaround. It felt like pure magic.

Lesson 3: You Can Achieve the "Unachievable"

Remember your first race? For me, on my first marathon I hit the wall at mile 20 (32 km), feeling like death, swearing that anything beyond 26.2 (42.2 km) was impossible. We've all been there in one way or another. But here's the thing about "impossible." It's usually just another word for "I haven't done it yet."

Through consistent training, those mental barriers started crumbling. First, 28 miles (45 km) became possible. Then 35 miles (56 km). Then 50 miles (80 km). When I decided to attempt 100 miles (161 km), sure, it felt like a massive leap into the unknown. But that's exactly where the magic happens.

Here's what I want you to understand: That big, scary goal you're thinking about? The one that makes your stomach flip when you consider it? That's not your limit. That's your invitation.

So here's my challenge to you: Take that goal that feels just out of reach, the one you've been saying "maybe someday" to. Make it your "Why not now?" Whether it's your first 10K race, a sub-6/5/4/3-hour marathon attempt, or yes, even 100 miles (161 km), declare it. Own it. Then start moving toward it.

Your impossible is waiting. What are you going to do about it?

Chapter Summary

- Pace patiently from the start. Conservative early pacing prevents the brutal slowdown that comes from starting too aggressively in ultra-distances.
- Fuel strategically and don't underestimate nutrition's importance. Simple fixes like caffeine can provide miraculous energy turnarounds.
- Mental barriers that seem "impossible" are often just "I haven't done it yet." Tackle big dreams with consistent small steps to unlock breakthroughs.

Recommended Resources

To help you turn the insights from this book into real-world results, I've created several free resources that you can access right away:

Running Toolkit | florisgierman.com/gift

Download this bundle of tools, including a Race Day Success Checklist, Nutrition Guide, and Training Workbook to help apply the book's lessons in real life.

Weekly Newsletter | florisgierman.com/subscribe

Every week, I send out a short, actionable email packed with insights to enhance your running performance and overall health. Expect tips, gear recommendations, training hacks and what I've been learning and testing that week.

My Favorite Gear | florisgierman.com/resources

Discover the gear and tools I personally use and recommend. From footwear and apparel to nutrition, hydration and recovery essentials, this is your go-to resource. You'll also get exclusive discounts from our brand partners.

The Extramilest Show | extramilest.com/podcast

Explore my conversations with world-class athletes, coaches and experts. All episodes are available here, along with show notes and direct links to YouTube and podcast platforms.

Connect on other channels:

Stay inspired, motivated and informed by following along on these platforms:

- **YouTube:** youtube.com/florisgierman
- **Instagram:** instagram.com/florisgierman
- **Strava:** strava.com/athletes/florisgierman

Top 25 Extramilest Podcasts

My Extramilest Podcast journey began in 2015. It started as a humble YouTube channel that now reaches millions of runners worldwide and has amassed more than 12 million combined YouTube views and podcast downloads.

I wanted to share the episodes that have resonated most deeply with our community. These rankings represent the most impactful conversations based on total reach, while accounting for release timing to ensure fair comparison between newer and established episodes.

These episodes showcase conversations that have genuinely changed how people approach their running. Whether you're looking to optimize your training, prevent injuries or simply find more joy in your miles, these episodes offer invaluable insights for runners at every level.

The Most Impactful Conversations from Extramilest Podcasts, Based on Research

#47: Eliud Kipchoge's Advice to Improve Your Running, For Non-Elites	extramilest.com/47
#51: Kilian Jornet's Advice to Improve Your Running	extramilest.com/51
#3: Dr. Phil Maffetone Interview on Heart Rate Training, Nutrition and Recovery	extramilest.com/3
#50: Dr. Stephen Seiler on 80/20 Training	extramilest.com/50
#88: Courtney Dauwalter's Advice to everyday runners	extramilest.com/88
#97: Taylor Knibb's Advice To Improve Your Running, Cycling and Swimming	extramilest.com/97
#67: Low Heart Rate Training Guide with Floris Gierman	extramilest.com/67
#16: Race Faster by Training Slower, with 2:28 Marathoner Josh Sambrook	extramilest.com/16
#83: Kipchoge's Top Running Tips for Athletes of All Levels	extramilest.com/83
#63: Low heart rate training with 2:44 marathoner Wissam Kheir	extramilest.com/63
#54: Ryan Hall on Strength Training for Runners	extramilest.com/54
#64: Beat The Wall! Race Day Nutrition with Andy Blow	extramilest.com/64
#38: Matt Fitzgerald on 80/20 Running & Running the Dream!	extramilest.com/38
#58: How to run healthy & strong, with Dr. Mark Cucuzzella (2:24 marathoner)	extramilest.com/58
#48: Sally McRae on Achieving Your Goals	extramilest.com/48
#25: Danny Dreyer from Chi Running on Energy Efficiency and Injury Prevention	extramilest.com/25
#56: Massive Running Improvements, 3:34 to 2:27 Marathon with Gareth King	extramilest.com/56
#39: Improve Your Running and Health with Dr. Phil Maffetone	extramilest.com/39
#33: Kofuzi on MAF Heart Rate Training for Running	extramilest.com/33
#52: Kilian Jornet Round 2, Training Advice & UTMB Lessons	extramilest.com/52
#80: Lawrence van Lingen, Massive Running Improvements	extramilest.com/80
#28: Misconceptions about MAF Training, by Floris Gierman	extramilest.com/28
#35: MAF Training Frustrations and Improvements, with Kathryn and Jennifer Geyer	extramilest.com/35
#5: Mark Allen on Heart Rate Training and Racing	extramilest.com/5
#96: How Eric Floberg Cut 86 Minutes: 3:59 to 2:33 Marathon	extramilest.com/96

Final Thoughts

What an incredible privilege it's been to host these conversations over the years. If you're new to the Extramilest podcast, I hope this collection serves as a roadmap to discovering episodes that might transform your running journey. For longtime listeners, perhaps this is an invitation to revisit episodes that sparked something in you the first time around.

The heart of this podcast has always been about helping everyday runners achieve extraordinary things through smarter, more sustainable approaches to training. As we continue this journey together, I remain committed to bringing you conversations that challenge conventional wisdom, inspire new possibilities and help you become the strongest, healthiest runner you can be.

Thank you for being part of this community. Here's to many more miles and meaningful conversations ahead!

Conclusion: Advice to My Younger Self

One of the questions I love to ask my guests on *The Extramilest Show* is "If you could go back in time, what advice would you give to your younger self just starting out in running or on their journey to better health?" Now it's my turn to answer that question.

The Artist Within the Runner

We begin with everything: every training, every race completed, every challenge we overcame. This is our source material. Running isn't merely physical movement; it's a creative act. With each run, you're composing a narrative about who you are becoming. Your body is the instrument; your mind, the composer.

Awareness Is Your Superpower

The difference between an average runner and an extraordinary one isn't merely talent, it's awareness. Notice how you really feel; how your feet strike the ground. Notice your controlled breathing. Observe the subtle sensations that signal when to push and when to ease back. This expanded awareness isn't something you force. It's something you allow to happen, a presence with what is happening in the eternal now of your run. Take moments throughout your day to tune in to yourself. Breathwork, meditation and journaling are powerful tools for this.

Tiny Changes, Remarkable Results

The path to extraordinary results is built by tiny, consistent actions. Improving by 1% isn't particularly notable and sometimes isn't even noticeable, but it can be far more meaningful in the long run. These 1% improvements over long enough time end up with extraordinary progress. You get what you repeat. Your running ability is a lagging measure of your training habits. Your health is a lagging measure of your eating habits.

Be Patient with the Plateau

In the early stages of any quest, there are often challenges. You expect linear progress, and it's frustrating when changes seem ineffective during the first weeks or months.

People make small changes, fail to see tangible results, and quit. But habits need to persist long enough to break through this plateau. When you finally break through, people will call it an overnight success. But you know it's the work you did long ago that makes today's leap possible. Think long-term, and be patient.

Do the Work, but Stay Flexible

There's no getting around it: You have to put in the work. That means running, eating well and getting enough sleep. But life happens, and sometimes your plan doesn't go perfectly. And that's okay. Being too rigid can lead to burnout. If you have to cut a run short or miss a workout, don't beat yourself up over it. Prioritize recovery, because that's where the magic happens. In the long run, being flexible when things come up will keep you more consistent than forcing every workout to happen, no matter what.

Build the Right Support System

Over the past 20 years, I've invested over $50,000 hiring coaches and experts to accelerate my progress in running, health and life. Guidance from experienced coaches can save you years of trial and error. A thriving community of like-minded people can also fast-track your progress and keep you accountable. My advice to my younger self would be to hire coaches and experts earlier in my journey.

Remember Why You Started

At its core, running isn't about achieving goals or impressing others. It's about discovering the artist within, the part of you that creates not because you have to but because you get to.

Each run is an act of self-expression, an opportunity to commune with something larger than yourself. Ultimately, breakthroughs happen when you grasp the big picture and recognize how holistic training principles apply not just to running but to every aspect of your life. The universe is only as large as our perception of it. When we cultivate our awareness through running, we expand the universe.

The path of the runner, like the path of the artist, is one of continuous evolution. There is no arrival, only the ongoing practice of being fully present with each step, each breath, each moment.

What It All Means: The Practice of Becoming

Beyond all the practical advice about training and technique lies a deeper truth about happiness and becoming.

The Choice

Happiness is a decision before it is a feeling. There are plenty of reasons you can be one of the happiest people alive.

You simply decide: I will be someone who figures this out. And then, step by step, you do.

Grace as Foundation

Give yourself grace. You are doing the best you can with what you have. This is not lowering standards. This is choosing clarity over punishment.

Some training days will be easy. Some runs will flow. At other times, life will interfere. This is not failure. This is the human experience.

When you stop performing for invisible judges and run for the simple joy of movement, you discover something beyond achievement. You discover presence.

The Courage to Be Different

Exceptional people do not fit in. This is what makes them exceptional.

When others question your changes, hear it as recognition of your growth. Most people haven't seen real transformation, so they don't know how to talk about it.

The runner who chooses solitude at dawn and who slows down when culture demands speed understands something about authenticity that conformity cannot teach.

Surrender

Running teaches the art of letting go. When you release the need to prove something with every stride, and train by feel rather than ego, you learn that forcing is just fear in disguise.

This letting go opens us, not to weakness, but to wonder. To what we cannot control.

The Unknown Territory

Everything valuable emerges from uncertainty. What feels safe is often just a familiar limitation.

Each run begins with a step into the unknown. Will your body respond? Will your mind quiet? Will you discover something new about who you are becoming?

This uncertainty is not the enemy. It is the birthplace of possibility.

The Practice

Happiness is not a finish line. It is the ongoing choice to align with what makes you feel most alive, rather than what makes you look most acceptable.

You can live with this natural authenticity. Trust the process. Offer yourself grace. And return to who you've always been, beneath all the noise of who you thought you had to be.

Need Extra Support?

Transform Your Running with Expert Coaching and Community Guidance

If you'd like additional guidance beyond this book, I've created resources that go deeper into these concepts in our Personal Best Running Coaching Program at PBprogram.com.

Perfect for:

- **Beginner Runners** who want a solid foundation and wish to avoid common training mistakes
- **Intermediate Runners** seeking structured plans to break through performance plateaus
- **Advanced Athletes** aiming to optimize their training and achieve new personal records
- **Runners Recovering** from Injuries looking for a sustainable and safe approach
- **Busy Professionals** needing flexible training plans that fit demanding schedules
- **Runners of All Ages** from 5K enthusiasts to ultramarathoners (our members range from 20 to 80+)

Why Join the PB Program?

- **Train Smarter, Not Harder:** Understand the purpose behind each workout, optimize your intensity-recovery balance and replace guesswork with science-backed methods.
- **Get Expert Coaching:** Receive guidance from RRCA-certified coaches through weekly live Q&A sessions addressing your specific questions.
- **Use Flexible Training Plans:** Access 20+ customizable training schedules that adapt to your life and goals, from base-building to race-specific preparation.
- **Join a Supportive Community:** Connect with 1,000+ like-minded runners who understand your journey and help keep you accountable.
- **Race with Confidence:** Develop proven race day strategies, learn effective pacing and avoid common pitfalls like "hitting the wall."

What You'll Get When You Join

- **Lifetime Access** to the complete PB Program
- **Step-by-Step Video Training** (20+ hours of my best content not available elsewhere)
- **Flexible Training Schedules** for all experience levels (Zone 2/MAF, base building, high intensity)
- **Weekly Live Coaching Calls** with Floris and other PB coaches
- **Supportive Online Community** of 1,000+ runners via private Facebook and Strava groups
- **Comprehensive Workbooks** to track your progress
- **Accountability Challenges** to maintain motivation
- **Race Preparation Guidance** for events from 5K to ultramarathon
- **60-Day Money-Back Guarantee**—try it risk-free!

Proven Results from Members:

- *"I've been literally in tears since I discovered this program. Everything about it makes me love running again! I plan to fight turning 50 all the way!"* —Missy Schmit

- *"Consistent PBs across all distances: 5K, 10K, half and full marathons. At 51, I'm in the best shape of my life."* —Daniel Edwards

- *"Completed 1,000 km injury-free, doubling my typical annual mileage. Incredible program!"* —Garth Boyd

- *"The best money spent to learn how to run in the best possible way. My days are more and more energetic, and I can quickly improve my aerobic condition."* —Emanuele Paris

- *"I'm a busy 50-year-old mom, and Floris and the PB Program have tremendously improved my fitness. This program benefits everyone, fast or slow."* —Tina Osborne

- *"Improved my 5K from 27:49 to 24:07 and my marathon from 4:10 to 3:54 within 5 months."* —Jonathan Pitayanukul, 64

- *"I improved my half-marathon PR by 26 minutes, from 2:32 to 2:06 on a hilly course. Highly recommended!"* —Ken Nguyen, 53

- *"Dropped 32 minutes off my marathon PR in just 6 months. This program is a treasure trove of low heart rate running wisdom!"* —Hyduke Noshadi, 40

Try the PB Program Risk-Free for 60 Days

The PB Program has helped thousands of runners train smarter, avoid injuries and achieve breakthrough performances. If you follow the program and don't see improvements within 60 days, you'll receive a full refund.

Join today at PBprogram.com

Acknowledgments

A massive thanks to my dear friend and mentor Lawrence van Lingen. Your guidance transformed my running and my life more than words can convey. Thank you for teaching me to move freely and discover flow states, and for reminding me always to be my authentic self. I'm honored by your thoughtful foreword.

Most importantly, thank you to my wife, Jen, whose patience and unwavering support made this book possible. Your strength in holding down the home front while I balanced full-time work with creating podcasts during early mornings, late nights and weekends has been monumental. Thanks for always being there, enabling me to train, race and complete the World Marathon Majors all over the world.

To my daughters, Sadie and Zoey, thank you for filling every run together with wonder and adventure, from double-stroller expeditions to nighttime trail explorations with headlamps. We never just "went for a run"; we always "went on adventures" looking for rocks and wildlife. Your creativity, joy and boundless curiosity make every moment brighter. Your births inspired me profoundly to become the strongest, healthiest and most present version of myself. Being your dad is my greatest joy.

Thank you to my parents, Hans and Ivon, and my sister, Janneke, for inspiring me to run my first local 5K at age eight. Watching you enjoy your runs planted seeds I only now fully appreciate in my forties. I finally understand why you did those funny-looking mobility exercises that made my sister and me laugh so hard as kids.

Thank you, Dr. Phil Maffetone, for introducing me to low heart rate training at such a pivotal moment in my life. Your holistic perspective on training, nutrition, sleep, stress and mindset fundamentally changed how I approach not only running but life itself.

Deep appreciation goes to my first running coaches, Jimmy Dean Freeman and Kate Martini Freeman. Your encouragement and belief in me helped me realize that I could dream bigger, and run farther, than I had ever imagined possible.

Thanks to my incredible business partners at Path Projects: Scott Bailey, Erich Frey, Brian Rather and Billy Yang. Building our running apparel company together has been a wild, rewarding adventure, and I'm grateful to share this journey with such an inspiring team.

Special recognition to Duc Tran, Jozef Matyasek, Amelia Vrabel, Scott Frye, Tim Garrett, Lewis Wu, Philip Bader, Bob Harpole, Russ Kemp, Steven Young, Dan Rawson, Troy Eckert, Karyn Lewandowski, Ashly Winchester, Ben Edusei, Kyle Long, Frank Sanchez, Andy Blow, Eric Chevalley, Matthew Crooker, Louise Kim, Charles Kim, Tonia Maddock, Leanne Dare, Matt Meadows, Geoff Rowley, Damien Gomez, Jack Rosenfeld, Don Reichelt, Ryan Kingman, Herm Golbach, Sander Op Den Dries, Mark van der Noord, Vincent de Vogel, Iain Jones, Andrew Cannon, Kerry Ward, Sam Monac, Dan Figur, Paul Sinclair and David Villalobos. Each of you has contributed to my growth, personally and professionally.

My deepest thanks to all listeners of *The Extramilest Show*. Your 20,000+ comments and messages have been a source of inspiration and motivation. Producing the podcast has truly been a labor of love, and your feedback and support mean everything to me. The heart of this work has always been about helping everyday runners achieve extraordinary things through smarter, more sustainable approaches to training.

A heartfelt thank you to all members of the PB Program. Getting to know you through our online community, weekly Zoom calls and shared race experiences worldwide has enriched my life immensely. Witnessing your growth and positive transformations beyond running keeps me inspired every day. You've created such a supportive and uplifting community.

Also, I want to extend my deepest gratitude to every guest on *The Extramilest Show*. Your willingness to share your wisdom and practical lessons forms the very heart of this book. Each conversation has been an immense privilege and a source of endless inspiration. In alphabetical order:

Mark Allen, Marco Altini, Bobby Barker, William Barth, John Birtchet-Sharpe, Zach Bitter, Andy Blow, Michael Brandt, Bill Callahan, Dr. Rangan Chatterjee, Jason Cherriman, Matt Choi, Kara Collier, Dr. Mark Cucuzzella,

Brent Cunningham, Larisa Dannis, Courtney Dauwalter, Jimmy Dean Freeman, Jay Dicharry, Julianne Dickerson, Jessica Dorsey, Danny Dreyer, Ben Edusei, Daniel Edwards, Charlie Engle, Martinus Evans, Ayako Fackenthal, Astrid Feyer, Matt Fitzgerald, Erich Floberg, Matteo Franceschetti, Kate Martini Freeman, Don Freeman, Scott Frye, Jennifer Geyer, Kathryn Geyer, Tawnee Gibson, Gurpreet Gill, Ryan Hall, Chris Hauth, Nate Helming, Wim Hof, Andy Hooks, Andrea Hudson, Nicki Hugie, Danny Huibregtse, Alex Hutchinson, Kilian Jornet, Jennifer Kellett, Wissam Kheir, Gareth King, Eliud Kipchoge, Taylor Knibb, Kofuzi, Pete Kostelnick, Aaron Kubala, Brendan Leonard, Ash Lewis, Walter Liniger, Kyle Long, Liam Lonsdale, Sean Lee, Arthur Lydiard, Dr. Phil Maffetone, Todd Marentette, Patrick McKeown, Sally McRae, Heidi Moreno, Jay Motley, Meaghan Murray-Neuberger, Greg Nance, Thomas Neuberger, Gwen Ostrosky, Michael Ovens, Jeroen Pieter van der Vliet, Susan Piver, Kelley Puckett, Robbe Reddinger, Tim Rowberry, Calvin Sambrook, Josh Sambrook, Jennifer Schmidt, Dr. Stephen Seiler, Albert Shank, Jeffrey Silver, Triathlon Taren, Duc Tran, Kasper van der Meulen, Lawrence van Lingen, Amelia Vrabel, Dr. Scott Vrzal, Jonathan Walton, Scott Warr, Maria Lurenda Westergaard, Kyle Whalum, Andy Wheatcroft, Ryan Whited.

Last but not least, thank you for being part of this journey with me. Whether you're reading these words, listening to the podcast or watching on YouTube, you are the heart of this community. Your stories inspire me, your questions challenge me, and your feedback reminds me why I do this work. Here's to the meaningful miles we've shared and the many more ahead!

Much love,
Floris Gierman

Glossary

When discussing technical or physiological concepts in this book, I have tried to use the simplest language wherever possible to ensure clarity and readability. In some cases, I have not always included definitions or explanations in the text, trusting that many readers will have at least a basic understanding of the context. This brief glossary provides additional information about key concepts, ideas and topics addressed in the book for those who might need or want them.

80/20 principle
A training philosophy where 80% of workouts are done at low intensity and 20% at high intensity.

Achilles
A tendon connecting the calf muscles to the heel bone, commonly stressed in running.

active recovery
Low-intensity exercise performed after intense activity to promote recovery.

adaptations
Physiological changes in the body in response to consistent training, such as improved endurance and muscle strength.

aerobic base
The foundation of cardiovascular fitness, built through low-intensity endurance training.

aerobic reset
A period of exclusive low-intensity aerobic training to rebuild the aerobic system and correct imbalances.

aerobic system
The energy system that uses oxygen to convert fat and carbohydrates into energy during sustained efforts.

anaerobic metabolism
: The energy system that generates power without oxygen, used during short, intense efforts.

anorexia
: An eating disorder characterized by self-imposed starvation and excessive weight loss, detrimental to performance and health.

anterior chain
: The group of muscles on the front of the body, including the hip flexors and quadriceps, important for running posture.

biomechanics
: The study of movement mechanics, important for efficient and injury-free running.

bulimia
: An eating disorder involving binge eating followed by purging, harmful to both health and athletic performance.

cadence
: The number of steps a runner takes per minute, often linked to running efficiency and injury prevention.

calorie
: Unit of energy provided by food, essential for fueling training and recovery.

capillaries
: Tiny blood vessels that deliver oxygen and nutrients to muscles and remove waste products.

carbohydrate
: A macronutrient and primary energy source for runners, stored in muscles and liver as glycogen.

cardiovascular system
: The heart and blood vessels that transport oxygen and nutrients throughout the body.

CO_2 tolerance
: The body's ability to tolerate higher levels of carbon dioxide, often improved through breath training.

cognitive behavioral therapy for insomnia (CBTI)
: A structured, evidence-based treatment for sleep issues, beneficial for recovery.

continuous glucose monitoring
A method to track blood sugar levels in real time, useful for nutrition and energy management.

electrolyte
Minerals like sodium and potassium essential for hydration and muscle function during endurance activities.

Epsom salts
Magnesium sulfate used in baths to help relax muscles and reduce soreness.

fartlek
A form of unstructured interval training combining periods of fast running with slower recovery jogs.

fat oxidation
The process by which the body uses fat as fuel, particularly during lower-intensity exercise.

flexion
A bending movement that decreases the angle between two body parts, important in running mechanics.

flow state
A mental state of deep focus and immersion, often experienced during optimal running performance.

fructose
A simple sugar found in fruit; used in some sports nutrition for quick energy.

glucose
A simple sugar that is a key energy source for muscles during running.

glycogen
The stored form of glucose in muscles and liver, used as fuel during prolonged exercise.

habit stacking
A behavior strategy that builds new habits by attaching them to existing routines.

hip flexors
Muscles that lift the thigh toward the torso, critical for running stride and posture.

hyponatremia
   A dangerous drop in blood sodium levels, often caused by excessive fluid intake during endurance events.

insulin sensitivity
   How responsive cells are to insulin; improved with regular aerobic exercise and beneficial for energy use.

intensity discipline
   The practice of staying within prescribed effort zones to maximize training benefits and avoid burnout.

intercostal muscles
   Muscles between the ribs that support breathing, particularly important during high-intensity running.

intermittent fasting
   An eating pattern that alternates periods of eating with fasting, sometimes used for metabolic benefits.

intervals
   Training sessions with repeated bouts of high-intensity running followed by recovery periods.

IT bands
   Iliotibial bands; connective tissues running along the outer thigh, often implicated in running injuries.

Karvonen Formula
   A method to calculate target heart rate using resting and maximum heart rate for individualized training.

lactate threshold
   The intensity of exercise at which lactate starts to accumulate in the blood, key for endurance performance.

lactic acid
   A byproduct of anaerobic metabolism that contributes to muscle fatigue during intense exercise.

MAF Method
   Maximum Aerobic Function Method; a heart-rate-based approach to improve aerobic efficiency and fat burning.

meditation
   A mental practice that enhances focus, reduces stress and can support recovery and performance.

metabolic pathways
Biochemical routes the body uses to convert food into energy, including aerobic and anaerobic systems.

mitochondria
Cellular structures that generate energy from oxygen and nutrients, crucial for endurance.

naked carbs
Carbohydrates eaten without protein, fat or fiber, which can lead to blood sugar spikes.

PB
Personal Best; the fastest time an individual has achieved for a specific running distance.

pelvic floor
Muscles at the base of the pelvis that support posture and stability during running.

polarized training
A method where most training is done at low intensity with some very high-intensity sessions.

PR
Personal Record; synonymous with Personal Best, used to track progress in race times.

progression runs
Runs that gradually increase in pace, used to simulate race conditions and improve stamina.

reactive hypoglycemia
A drop in blood sugar after eating, potentially affecting energy levels during running.

stride
The length and rhythm of a runner's step, influencing efficiency and speed.

Super Shoes
High-tech running shoes with carbon plates and foam designed to improve performance.

sympathetic nervous system
The part of the nervous system responsible for the fight-or-flight response, activated during intense exercise.

tempo runs
> Steady runs at a "comfortably hard" pace to improve lactate threshold and endurance.

training intensity
> The level of effort or exertion in a workout, typically measured by heart rate or perceived effort.

training volume
> The total amount of running over a period, usually measured in miles or hours per week.

two-minute rule
> A strategy to overcome procrastination by committing to just two minutes of activity to build momentum.

vagus nerve
> A nerve involved in parasympathetic control of the heart and digestion, associated with recovery and stress regulation.

vision board
> A visual tool displaying goals and aspirations to motivate and focus training efforts.

vitamin D deficiency
> A lack of vitamin D, which can affect bone health and energy levels, particularly in endurance athletes.

VO_2 max
> The maximum amount of oxygen the body can use during intense exercise; a key indicator of aerobic fitness.

www.ingramcontent.com/pod-product-compliance
Lightning Source LLC
Chambersburg PA
CBHW080539030426
42337CB00024B/4797